YOGA

FOR

RUNNERS AND CYCLISTS

**10-minutes Poses And Techniques
To Improve Your Performance**

Roy A. Starr

TABLE OF CONTENTS

CHAPTER 1: Introduction

A synopsis of yoga

CHAPTER 2:   Yoga For Cyclists And Runners:

- Developing Synergy to Perform at Your Best
- The Significance of yoga
- Diverse Benefits of yoga

CHAPTER 3. Understanding Runners' and Cyclists' Body

- Anatomy and Physiology

 - Runner's anatomy basics

 - Cyclist's anatomy basics

- Common Injuries in Running and Cycling

- Common running injuries and recovery tips

- Common cycling injuries and recovery tips

CHAPTER 4. Fundamentals of yoga practice

- A Comprehensive Look

  - The Philosophical Bases:

  - Getting started with yoga at home

- Breath Awareness and Control

  - Techniques for breath awareness in yoga

  - Breathing exercises for runners and cyclists

CHAPTER 5. Yoga Poses for Runners

- Yoga Stretching Exercises:

CHAPTER 6. Yoga Poses for Cyclists

- Pre-ride Stretching Routine
  - Yoga stretches for cyclists before riding
  - Warm-up Cycling Poses Before Yoga

- Posits For Post-ride Recovery
  - Yoga poses for recovery after cycling
  - Cool-down yoga routine for cyclists

- Poses for Balance and Core Strength
  - Yoga poses to improve balance for cyclists
  - Core-strengthening yoga poses for cyclists

CHAPTER 7. Breathwork for Endurance

- Pranayama Techniques for Runners
  - Breathwork for endurance run
  - Pranayama for improved running performance

- Cyclists' Pranayama Techniques

  - Breathing exercises for cycling stamina

  - Pranayama for enhanced cycling endurance

CHAPTER 8: Consciousness And Mental Strength

- Yoga as a Stress Reduction Technique

  - Meditation and yoga as stress relievers

  - Mindfulness Exercises Among Cyclists And Runners

- Runners' and Cyclists' Endurance Mental Strategies

  - Mental resilience techniques for runners

  - Techniques For Staying Focused On Lengthy Journeys

CHAPTER 9: Nutrition and Hydration

- Supporting Your Body with Proper Nutrition

- Nutrition advice for runners and cyclists

- Fueling your body for endurance activities

- Hydration Tips for Endurance Activities

- Hydration strategies for runners and cyclists

- Importance of staying hydrated during long rides

CHAPTER 10: Recovery Strategies

- The Value Of Sleep And Rest

- Benefits Of Rest For Recovery In Cyclists And Runners

- Techniques for having a quality sleep for Cyclists and Runners:

- Stretching and Self-Massage Methods

- Ways In Which You Can Do Self-Massage Effectively:

- Stretching exercises to improve healing and flexibility:

CHAPTER 11: Building a Sustainable Yoga Routine

- Integrating Yoga into Training Plans

- Incorporating yoga into running training plans

- Adding yoga to cycling training schedules

- Creating a Personalized Practice

- Personalized yoga routines for runners and cyclists

- Advantages Of An Eco-friendly Yoga Program for Cyclists and Runners:

- Essential Elements of a Long-Term Yoga Practice:

No part of this book may be reproduced or transmitted in any form or by any electronic or mechanical means, including photocopying, recording, or information storage and retrieval systems, without the express permission of the publisher, 2024. All rights reserved by Roy A. Starr

CHAPTER 1

A SYNOPSIS OF YOGA

The age-old, highly respected discipline of yoga offers anyone looking for a comprehensive approach to wellbeing a timeless manual. With its origins in the Sanskrit word "yuj," which means to merge or join, the name "yoga" dates back to ancient India. This etymology encapsulates the essence of yoga, which emphasizes interconnectivity and harmony while going beyond the boundaries of physical activity to create a union between the individual self and the global consciousness.

Yoga's historical fabric is a complex tapestry made of strands from many philosophical and spiritual traditions. The Vedas, ancient Indian texts that provide a conceptual framework for comprehending life, lay the groundwork for it. A wide range of yoga styles and methods have been developed throughout time as a result of the emergence of different schools of thought and practices.

The "Yoga Sutras," which date to around 200 BC and are credited to the sage Patanjali, represent a significant turning point in the codification of yoga. The teachings of Patanjali, which are condensed into this ancient work, provide a methodical and thorough manual for practicing yoga. According to the sutras, yoga has eight branches: asanas (physical postures), pranayama (breath control), concentration, meditation, and ethical principles (yamas and niyamas). Together, these limbs provide a path that leads to spiritual enlightenment and self-realization.

Yoga is now a worldwide phenomenon that has crossed cultural barriers in the contemporary period. It offers a range of techniques, from the physically demanding and energetic Ashtanga and Vinyasa to the healing and contemplative Yin and Hatha practices, adapting to a variety of lifestyles. Modern yoga goes beyond the physical poses and combines mindfulness, stress relief, and general wellbeing, which appeals to those who want a holistic approach to health.

The many advantages of yoga have been highlighted by scientific studies, which support the practice's beneficial effects on mental clarity, emotional stability, and physical health. Yoga is well known for its ability to improve people of all ages and backgrounds, from lowering tension and anxiety to increasing strength and flexibility.

In the next chapters, we will dig into practical applications, explore the philosophical underpinnings of yoga, and uncover the deep wisdom that is ingrained in this age-old practice. Every chapter will act as a starting point for comprehending and adopting yoga as a complete way of life, providing guidance for anyone looking for a means to achieve balance, inner serenity, and self-discovery.

CHAPTER 2

YOGA FOR CYCLISTS AND RUNNERS:

- **Developing Synergy to Perform at Your Best**

Yoga is a comprehensive method that goes beyond conventional fitness regimens for bikers and runners. It functions as a versatile toolkit that addresses certain issues endurance athletes experience. Yoga becomes a transforming practice for maximising performance and avoiding injuries via a mix of dynamic conditioning, flexibility development, strength growth, core engagement, and breath awareness. It is an essential tool for athletes looking for a well-rounded and durable training regimen because of its versatility on different types of terrain, emphasis on joint health, and effective recuperation techniques. Yoga for runners and cyclists is essentially a technique that unlocks the potential for prolonged peak performance in the realm of endurance sports by fostering a harmonious connection between body and mind.

- **The Significance of yoga:**

1. Injury Avoidance with Holistic Exercise:

Yoga offers a comprehensive approach to conditioning, targeting the stabilizing muscles as well as the main muscle groups, which are sometimes disregarded. Running and cycling are repetitive sports; therefore, this thorough training lessens the likelihood of frequent ailments.

2. Unlocking Range of Motion and Flexibility: Yoga's many stretches help increase flexibility, which helps runners and cyclists maintain their ideal range of motion. This flexibility helps to minimize the risk of injuries, promote fluid movement, and avoid muscular imbalances.

3. Consolidating the bases: The many yoga positions work muscles in different ways, increasing strength and stamina. Yoga focuses on stabilizing muscles, strengthening the body's foundation, and improving general strength for prolonged performance, in addition to the main muscles utilized in running and cycling.

4. Stability of Core for Endurance: The foundation of endurance sports is a robust and solid core. Yoga's emphasis on core activation contributes to improved posture, increased stability, and a decreased risk of form deterioration due to exhaustion during prolonged periods of effort.

5. Using the Power of Breath:- Yoga's breath control technique, pranayama, is essential to maximizing respiratory efficiency. Learning to coordinate breath with movement is beneficial for endurance athletes since it has a major influence on energy management and endurance capability.

- **Diverse Benefits of yoga:**

1.Quicker Healing With Restorative Activities: Yoga's healing components provide the body with a safe haven for healing. Yoga sessions after training help athletes relax, ease tightness in their muscles, and speed up the healing process. This allows them to stick to a regular and efficient training regimen.

2. Strengthening Mental Capacity: Beyond the mat, yoga cultivates awareness, which helps endurance athletes develop mental toughness. Focus, attention, and the capacity to remain in the now are skills that

yoga imparts and are essential for overcoming the psychological obstacles that come with long-distance running and cycling.

3. Improving Coordination and Balance: Yoga's use of balancing postures improves coordination and proprioception, two essential skills for athletes negotiating a variety of terrains. The increased stability and spatial awareness that yoga practice fosters are especially helpful for trail runners and bikers.

4. Joint Health and Longevity: The soft stretches and motions of yoga promote joint mobility without adding to the strain on the joints, which helps maintain joint health and longevity. Yoga offers athletes a balance between the low-impact practice's ability to preserve their joints and the high-impact character of their activities.

5. Fostering an Intense Mind-Body Bond: Through yoga, one may develop a strong mind-body connection. Athletes experience an increase in body awareness, which fosters intuitive reactions to training loads and any warning signs. This improves general health and well-being and helps athletes avoid injuries.

Essentially, yoga goes beyond only physical fitness when it comes to the training regimens of cyclists and runners. It turns into a voyage of transformation where the body, mind, and breath are all in sync to achieve peak performance. Athletes may fully benefit from yoga by practicing consistently and consciously, creating a symbiotic connection that lasts far beyond the finish line.

CHAPTER 3

UNDERSTANDING RUNNERS' AND CYCLISTS' BODY

A. Runners' Body Anatomy and Physiology:

The anatomy and physiology of a runner's body are specially designed to fulfill the demands of sports activities, which encompass several systems and tissues that collaborate to provide effective and prolonged running. Let's examine each of the main points in detail:

1. Cardiovascular System:

Heart: The heart's function as the central pump is to pump oxygen-rich blood to the working muscles and return oxygen-depleted blood to the lungs for replenishment. Running improves cardiovascular health by fortifying and enhancing the heart's function. Frequent endurance exercise causes the heart to adapt by increasing cardiac output and stroke volume, which increases the amount of blood the organ pumps out with each beat.

Blood Vessels: Vasodilation, which is enhanced blood flow to muscles via running, causes blood vessels to dilate. Muscles have expanding capillaries that maximize the transport of nutrients and oxygen to enable the creation of energy. During extended activity, this adaptation increases the effectiveness of waste clearance and nutrition exchange.

2. **Respiratory System:**

Lungs: Running puts strain on the respiratory system and increases the need for oxygen intake in the lungs. The lungs adjust by expanding lung capacity and enhancing oxygen diffusion. This adaptation supports the increased oxygen demand during prolonged aerobic exertion by improving the efficiency of oxygen exchange in the alveoli.

Diaphragm and Intercostal Muscles: The diaphragm and intercostal muscles are essential for breathing. Running improves breathing patterns and endurance by strengthening these respiratory muscles. Stronger respiratory muscles are necessary to sustain regular breathing even under stressful conditions.

3. Muscles Of The Lower Extremities:

Leg Muscles: Major muscle groups used in running include the hamstrings, quadriceps, calf muscles, and hip flexors. During foot striking, these muscles contract regularly to move the body forward and absorb force. Muscle hypertrophy and increased endurance capability in these muscle groups are the results of endurance running.

Core Muscles: During running, the core stabilizes the body, promoting good biomechanics and balance. Maintaining posture, avoiding form breakdown due to fatigue, and maximizing energy transmission all depend on core strength. Power transmission from the lower to the upper body is facilitated by a strong core, which is necessary for effective running mechanics.

Joints: Running's repeated nature strains joints, especially the ankles, hips, and knees. Sufficient strength and flexibility exercises lessen the force on joints and lower the chance of injury. Running-related joint adaptations, such as increased synovial fluid production, support long-term joint health.

Connective Tissues: Tendons and ligaments are examples of connective tissues that bind muscles to bones. Running improves joint stability and general structural integrity by encouraging these connective tissues to adapt and become stronger. Gradual adaptation is helpful in preventing overuse injuries brought on by stress on the connective tissues.

4. Nervous System:

Motor Neurons: To start muscular contractions and regulate movement, running requires exact synchronization of motor neurons. Training improves neuromuscular networks, which improves running mechanics efficiency and coordination. For more fluid and economical movement, the nervous system adapts by improving motor unit recruitment and synchronization.

Proprioception: For running stability, the neural system's capacity to detect the body's spatial location is essential. Running on different types of terrain and balancing exercises improve proprioception. Enhancing proprioception lowers the chance of trips, slides, and falls during running by improving body awareness.

5. Endocrine System:

Adrenal Glands: Running long distances causes stress hormones like cortisol and adrenaline to be released more readily. Acute stress is a natural physiological reaction to running, but persistent stress may harm one's health and ability to recuperate. Maintaining a healthy hormonal balance is facilitated by controlling training loads, eating well, and using recuperation techniques.

Hormones: Endorphins, which are linked to mood elevation, and growth hormone, which is crucial for muscle repair and recovery, are released when one runs, and this has an impact on the balance of hormones. Stress reduction and elevated mood are two of the psychological advantages of running that are attributed to positive hormone reactions.

6. Systems Of Energy:

Aerobic System: The primary energy source for long-distance running is aerobic energy production, which uses oxygen to turn fats and carbs into energy. This system functions more efficiently with aerobic exercise, which increases mitochondrial density, improves oxygen consumption, and increases endurance.

Anaerobic System: Anaerobic energy pathways, which depend on stored energy sources without oxygen, are activated during sprinting or other intensive exertion. Running intervals and speed training help runners increase their anaerobic capacity. Adapting to different intensities during races requires the capacity to switch between anaerobic and aerobic energy systems with efficiency.

7. Immune System And Reproductive Systems:

Reproductive Hormones: Reproductive hormones may be impacted by intense training, especially in female runners. It's critical to keep hormone health, diet, and exercise load in balance. Female runners may have irregular menstrual cycles or hormonal imbalances, which calls for careful consideration of their general health and dietary habits.

Immune System: While intense training loads might momentarily inhibit the immune system, moderate exercise promotes immunological function. For runners to have a healthy immune system, proper recuperation, diet, and rest are crucial. By balancing the intensity of exercise with sufficient rest, one may lower the risk of disease by preventing immune system damage.

It is critical for runners to comprehend the complex interactions between these physiological and anatomical elements. A robust and effective running body is a result of customizing training plans to meet individual demands and include components like strength training, flexibility exercises, and recovery techniques.

- **Cyclist's Body Physiology and Anatomy: Discovering the Performance Mechanics.**

The demands of cycling are particular to the human body because it needs a precise balance between anatomical features and physiological responses. A thorough examination of the anatomy and physiology of cyclists reveals the complex processes that propel their endurance and performance.

1. **Cardiovascular System:**

Circulatory System and Heart: Cyclists' cardiovascular systems experience major changes. An increased stroke volume from endurance exercise enables the heart to pump more blood with each beat. This makes sure that muscles get oxygen efficiently, especially when combined with an increased heart rate.

Capillary Density: The muscles of cyclists often grow more capillaries, which improves the supply of nutrients and oxygen. This enhanced vascularity helps the body use energy more effectively and with greater endurance.

2. Respiratory System:

Lung Capacity: A healthy respiratory system is necessary for cycling. By increasing lung capacity, endurance training helps riders breathe in more oxygen and exhale carbon dioxide more effectively. Long rides require sustained effort, and this increased respiratory efficiency is essential.

Strengthening of the Diaphragm: Cyclists experience strengthening of this important respiratory muscle. This adaptation contributes to endurance and overall respiratory efficiency by helping to maintain a regular breathing pattern.

3. The Muscle System

Muscles of the Leg: The quadriceps, hamstrings, and calf muscles are the main muscles used in cycling. Training causes these muscles to hypertrophy and become more endurance-driven, enabling strong pedal strokes and prolonged, continuous effort.

Core Muscles: Stability and power transmission depend heavily on a robust core. To maintain proper posture, cyclists use their core muscles, particularly when climbing and sprinting. Frequent cycling improves core strength and lowers the chance of form breakdown due to fatigue.

4. Lower Limb Alignment in the Skeletal System Sustaining ideal lower-limb alignment requires proper bike fit. The femur and tibia in particular have been reinforced as part of the skeletal adaptations to endure the frequent demands of cycling.

Spinal Alignment: For comfort and effectiveness, the spine should be kept in a neutral posture. The spine adjusts to the pedaling position, and cyclists frequently gain improved flexibility in the lumbar and thoracic areas.

5. **Metabolic Adaptations:**

Energy Systems: Aerobic energy systems are mostly used in cycling. Endurance exercise boosts the body's capacity to use lipids as a fuel source, reserving glycogen for high-intensity activities. This metabolic flexibility is necessary for extended rides.

Glycogen Storage: Cyclists enhance glycogen storage in muscles and the liver through diet and exercise. This offers a quickly accessible energy supply during strenuous exertion and minimizes early weariness.

6. **Nervous System:**

Neuromuscular Coordination: Cycling involves precise neuromuscular coordination for effective pedal strokes. Cyclists acquire increased motor control and synchronization, avoiding energy waste and maximizing power production.

Proprioception: The repeated nature of cycling hones proprioception, the body's perception of position and movement. This heightened proprioception assists in balance and control, particularly vital during maneuvers and varied terrains.

In essence, the physiology and anatomy of cyclists undergo amazing modifications created by the demands of the activity. From cardiovascular improvements and muscular strength to metabolic efficiency, the cyclist's body transforms into a finely tuned machine, harmonizing with the mechanical subtleties of the bicycle for best performance on the road. Understanding these physiological and anatomical intricacies is crucial to both enhancing performance and guaranteeing the long-term well-being of cyclists.

- **Common Injuries in Running and Cycling:**

  - *Common Running Injuries And Recovery Tips*

1. Shin Splints:

Overuse, inappropriate footwear, or jogging on hard surfaces are the causes.

Preventive measures include increasing mileage gradually, using appropriate shoes, and strengthening your calf muscles. Using softer jogging surfaces might also lessen the impact.

2. Syndrome of Patellofemoral Pain (Runner's Knee):

Causes: overuse, muscular imbalances, and kneecap misalignment.
Prevention involves avoiding abrupt changes in training intensity, maintaining good running form, and strengthening the quadriceps and hip muscles. Activities for cross-training that don't put tension on the knee may also help.

3. Syndrome of the IT Band:

Causes: overuse or muscle imbalances causing the IT band to rub on the knee joint.
Preventive measures include frequent foam rolling, IT band strengthening and stretching activities, and avoiding sudden changes in running surfaces. Muscle imbalances may be addressed in the regimen by including lateral leg movements.

4. Plantar fasciitis:

Causes: Plantar fasciitis is brought on by excessive use or inappropriate footwear.
Prevention includes wearing supportive shoes, gradually increasing distance, and stretching the plantar fascia and calf on a regular basis. You may get relief by rolling your foot over a frozen water bottle.

- ***Common Cycling Injuries And Recovery Tips***

1. Lower back pain:

Causes: muscle imbalances, poor posture while riding, and poorly fitted bikes.
Preventive measures include making sure your bike fits properly, keeping your spine in a neutral posture, and doing core-strengthening activities. Tensions may be relieved by routinely stretching the hip flexors and lower back.

2. Pain in the knees:

Causes: overuse, misalignment, or improper bike fit. Prevention involves strengthening your hamstrings and quadriceps, adjusting the saddle height, and aligning your pedals and cleats correctly. Another way to lessen strain is to make sure your pedal stroke is smooth and steer clear of high gear ratios.

3. Problems with Urogenital Cycling:

Causes: riding posture or saddle design that puts pressure on the perineum.
Reduction: selecting a properly fitting saddle, putting on cushioned shorts, and modifying the height and tilt of the seat. Long rides might benefit from standing sometimes to release tension.

4. Syndrome of the Carpal Tunnel:

The cause is prolonged wrist strain from squeezing the handlebars.
Preventive measures include using ergonomic grips, modifying handlebar posture, and combining

wrist-strengthening workouts. During rides, shifting your hands around a lot might help spread the strain.

CHAPTER 4

FUNDAMENTALS OF YOGA PRACTICE

A Comprehensive Look:

Yoga is an ancient kind of physical exercise that has its roots in India and encompasses a comprehensive approach to well-being. Yoga, which has its roots in the Sanskrit word "yuj," which means to connect or combine, aims to bring the mind, body, and spirit into harmony. It is a multidimensional discipline that combines ethical concepts, physical postures, breath control, and meditation to provide a route towards inner calm, balance, and self-discovery.

- **The Philosophical Bases:**

1. The Yoga Eight Limbs:

The "Yoga Sutras," which are ascribed to the philosopher Patanjali, are the major texts of yogic philosophy. This ancient book describes the eight limbs of yoga and offers a methodical framework for leading a meaningful life. The limbs include concentration, breathing exercises (pranayama), physical postures (asanas), ethical precepts (yamas and niyamas), and meditation, which lead to the ultimate state of enlightenment (samadhi).

2. Nyamas and Yamas:

- Yoga's first two limbs, the yamas and niyamas, serve as its ethical cornerstone. Yamas include ethical precepts like honesty (satya) and nonviolence (ahimsa), while niyamas concentrate on individual practices like self-control (tapas) and contentment (santosha).

Physical Practice (Asanas):

1. Asanas - Pose Positions:

- The most well-known feature of yoga are perhaps its asanas, or physical postures. These postures, which range from easy stretches to difficult inversions, are designed to develop balance, strength, and flexibility. Every posture has special advantages for the body and mind.

2. Flow and Sequencing:

In yoga lessons, postures are performed in a certain order to warm up the body, increase intensity, and calm down. Popular vinyasa technique places emphasis on the flow between postures, linking breath and movement.

Inhalation - (Pranayama):

1. Pranayama - Control of Breath:

- Conscious breath control is a requirement in pranayama. Numerous methods are used to improve respiratory function, soothe the mind, and channel energy, such as diaphragmatic breathing (deep belly breathing) and nadi shodhana (alternating nostril breathing).

2. Asynchrony of Breath Movement:

- One of the main concepts is breathing and movement coordination. By bridging the gap between the mental and physical parts of yoga, the breath helps practitioners become more attentive and stay in the present moment.

Cognitive Exercises:

1. Mindfulness and Concentration:

Yoga uses techniques to develop mental attention in addition to physical training. Meditating and other concentration skills will help you become more self-aware and calm down. The advantages of mindfulness meditation in particular have made it more popular.

2. Psycho-Physical Link:

- Yoga highlights how closely the mind and body are connected. Practitioners learn to listen to their bodies, develop intuition, and attend to their emotional and physical needs via mindful movement and breath awareness.

Wellness in All Aspects:

1. Asana-Based Yoga:

Asanas are an essential component of yoga, but the practice goes beyond poses. It includes integrating yogic ideas into everyday life for holistic well-being, as well as ethical and lifestyle choices.

2. The Philosophy of Yoga in Practice:

- Yoga practice transcends the mat and becomes a way of life. Practices like appreciation, compassion, and mindfulness on the mat translate into everyday life and relationships.

A timeless and ever-evolving practice, yoga encourages people to delve into the core of who they are, leading to a journey of balance, resilience, and self-discovery. The foundational elements of yoga provide a deep and transforming route toward comprehensive well-being, whether one chooses to explore the physical aspects of asanas, delve into breath control and meditation, or embrace the ethical ideals.

Comprehensive Study of the Foundations of Yoga Practice

A fundamental path toward overall well-being is revealed by yoga, an age-old practice that goes beyond the merely physical. We explore the foundations of yoga practice, which includes physical postures, awareness of breath, meditation, and moral precepts. These principles, which have their roots in traditional knowledge, provide those looking for more than simply strength and flexibility; they also offer a path toward a closer relationship with both the outside world and ourselves.

Principles of Mindful Movement:

Creative Alignment:

- Mindful alignment during asana exploration is fundamental to a yoga practice. Every pose becomes a canvas for self-discovery, from the centered Mountain Pose to the flowing Warrior sequences. A comprehensive relationship between the body and mind is fostered by alignment, which prevents injury and promotes a balanced flow of energy.

2. Breathe as the Enzyme:

- The practice of mindful breathing is the foundation of yoga. The power of breath may be accessed via pranayama methods like the balanced Nadi Shodhana or the oceanic Ujjayi breath. It turns into a rhythmic mentor that synchronizes with motion to provide a moving meditation that enhances mental clarity in addition to physical energy.

Creating a Strong Foundation:

1. Key Asanas Pose Positions:

- A robust practice starts with the basic asanas. These poses, which range from the centered Tadasana to the contemplative Child's Pose, develop physical stamina, flexibility, and body awareness. Gaining control over these positions builds a solid basis for more difficult exercises.

2. Warm regards from the sun (Surya Namaskar):

Sun Salutations are the foundation of the yoga practice; they are a dynamic sequence that captures the essence of yoga's sunlike vigor. Surya Namaskar is a comprehensive exercise that feeds the body and soul. It consists of a sequence of interrelated positions that transform into a dance of breath and movement, kindling the inner fire.

Meditation And Mindfulness Techniques:

1. Mindfulness in Action:

- Yoga is a journey that goes beyond static poses to include active awareness. The mind-body connection becomes more acutely conscious as practitioners progress through sequences, with each movement offering a chance for deep presence.

2. Teacher-led mindfulness and meditation:

- The basics also include practicing meditation to develop inner peace. The practice of yoga is enhanced by methods like mindfulness and loving-kindness meditation, which promote mental clarity, emotional equilibrium, and a steadfast connection to the present.

Ethical Living: Yamas and Niyamas:

1. Adhering to Moral Standards:

- Yoga is about living an ethical life; it isn't only for the mat. The principles of non-violence (ahimsa), contentment (santosha), and honesty (satya) provide a moral compass for practitioners to live virtuous and balanced lives. These are the yamas and niyamas.

Acceleration and Flexibility:

1. Personal Exploration:

Yoga is fundamentally a voyage of self-discovery. The principles encourage people to accept and value their own body modifications. Every exercise becomes a medium for introspection and self-revelation.

2. The Patience Art:

- Yoga's foundations are similar to the practice of patience. Development is a slow process rather than a quick fix. Transformations occur on the physical, mental, and emotional levels with regular practice. Yoga turns into a lifetime endeavour, a never-ending process of personal development.

In discovering the foundations of yoga, people set out on a deep journey that reaches beyond the mat and into the fabric of daily life. It involves self-exploration, conscious movement, moral behaviour, and the development of a peaceful life. Yoga is more than just an exercise program; it's a place where people may create their own personal blueprint for inner peace, wellbeing, and an unwavering connection to life's fundamental core. The foundations of yoga become a timeless guide on this journey of transformation as we breathe, move, and contemplate.

- **Beginner's Guide to Yoga: A Detailed Look at How to Begin Your Practice**

A beginner's path into yoga entails accepting a diverse range of practices aimed at improving mental, emotional, and physical well-being. Here we explore the fundamentals, which include starting practices, poses, alignment principles, and other important elements necessary for a meaningful and long-lasting practice of yoga.

1. Breath awareness is the first step:

-Exercise:

Start with basic breathing techniques. For the purpose of creating a conscious link between breath and movement, concentrate on deep belly breathing and progressively include methods such as Ujjayi breath (victorious breath).

-Purpose:

Developing mindful breathing establishes the groundwork for synchronizing breath with physical postures and sets the tone for your practice by encouraging calm.

2. Asanas for Beginners: Foundational Postures

Exercise: Begin with fundamental postures such Warrior I (Virabhadrasana I), Downward-Facing Dog (Adho Mukha Svanasana), and Mountain Pose (Tadasana). These poses increase flexibility, strengthen the body, and familiarize the practitioner with alignment fundamentals.

Purpose: Developing body awareness, strengthening muscles and joints, and laying the framework for increasingly difficult poses are the goals of foundational poses in yoga.

3. Principles of Safety and Effectiveness Alignment:

- Exercise: Give alignment close attention. Learn the correct alignment of your body in each posture, paying particular attention to details like joint placement, spinal neutrality, and activation of the necessary muscle groups.

Purpose: Proper alignment not only maximizes the benefits of the postures and minimizes strain or injury, but it also assures safety.

4. Sun Salutation - Flowing Sequences:

Practice: Make Sun Salutations (Surya Namaskar) a part of your daily regimen. Lunges, forward folds, and upward and downward-facing dog positions are among the poses that make up this dynamic sequence.

Sun Salutations serve the following purposes: -They increase cardiovascular health, boost stamina, and provide a complete, full-body exercise. They act as an intermediary between still stances and fluid movements.

5. Comprehending Yoga Equipment:

-Exercise: Become acquainted with standard yoga props such as bolsters, straps, and blocks. In order to ensure comfort and correct alignment, use these props to assist your practice, particularly if you're just starting out.

-Purpose: Props help practitioners achieve proper postures, accommodate individual variations in flexibility, and avoid strain while keeping the practice fun and accessible.

6. Traits for Mindfulness and Relaxation:

Exercise: Introduce guided meditation and other mindfulness and relaxation techniques, such as corpse pose (Savasana). These quiet times improve brain clarity, lower stress levels, and foster inner peace.

Purpose: By enhancing a comprehensive approach to wellbeing and strengthening the mind-body link, mindfulness practices support physical practice.

7. Advancing Gradually:

- Exercise: Advance according to your own speed. As your strength and flexibility increase, gradually work your way up to increasingly challenging postures and sequences. Accept the fact that your practice is a work in progress and have patience with yourself.

-Purpose: Gradual development promotes sustainability, avoids overstretching, and fosters an uplifting and inspiring yoga experience.

8. Paying Attention to Your Body:

-Exercise: Make it a habit to pay attention to your body's telling signs. When required, adjust positions, take pauses, and respect your boundaries. Respect your body's individuality and its reactions.

Purpose: Paying attention to your body develops a thoughtful and caring approach to your practice, increases self-awareness, and lowers the chance of injury.

Finally, When starting a yoga journey, a novice must embrace patience, curiosity, and a dedication to self-discovery. A strong foundation for a continuous and developing yoga practice is established by these fundamental techniques, postures, alignment concepts, and considerations. Enjoy every moment of this life-changing experience, welcome the process of learning, and let yoga develop into a nourishing and enlivening part of your being.

Beginning Yoga at Home: An All-Inclusive Guide

Taking up yoga at home is a fulfilling endeavour that offers convenience, flexibility, and an individualised approach to wellbeing. This comprehensive guide will help you develop and improve your at-home yoga practice, regardless of whether you're a newbie or coming back to the mat after a break.

1. Make a Special Place for It:

- Setup: Choose a peaceful, clutter-free space to do your practice. It should ideally have enough area for mobility and good ventilation. Think of including a blanket, a yoga mat, and any necessary accessories.

2. Select the Appropriate Gear:

-Yoga Mat: To ensure stability and comfort, spend your money on a high-quality yoga mat. It delineates your own zone while practising and offers a non-slip surface.

-Props: Get props like blocks, straps, or a bolster according to your requirements. They improve support, especially in the early going.

3. Please Choose Proper Clothes:

- Cozy Clothes: Dress in loose-fitting, airy clothes that don't restrict your mobility. This may improve your practicing experience overall and help you feel more comfortable.

4. Achieve sensible objectives:

Start Small: Whether you're brand-new to yoga or making a comeback, start with shorter practises. As your flexibility and strength improve, gradually increase the length and intensity of your practice.

Consistency: Try to be consistent rather than intense. To get the full range of yoga's benefits, consistency is essential.

5. Get Online Resources:

- Online courses: Look into websites that provide yoga courses with a teacher. A wide range of courses that accommodate varying levels, styles, and durations are offered by several platforms.

- Tutorials: Make use of tutorials or instructional videos that address alignment, breathing, and position breakdown. For home practitioners, these sites provide insightful advice.

6. Observe a Systematized Process:

Warming up gently is always the first step. To get your body ready for more strenuous poses, use exercises like shoulder stretches, neck rolls, and mild twists.

Asanas: Combine a variety of postures that work on various muscle groups in your asanas. As you develop your practice, go from basic postures to more challenging ones.

- Cool Down: After your practice, spend some time in relaxation postures such as child's pose or savasana.

7. Pranayama - Mindful Breathing:

Breath mindfulness: Include mindfulness of your breath in your routine. Concentrate on breathing steadily and deliberately, coordinating each breath with your actions.

-Pranayama Practices: Learn different pranayama methods such as breathing deep diaphragmatically or breathing through different nostrils. These encourage relaxation and expand lung capacity.

8. Pay Attention to Your Body:

-Adjustments for Yourself: Observe your body's reaction to every stance. Don't force yourself into pain or discomfort; instead, make the required modifications and utilize supports as needed.

-Change Positions: Adjust positions to suit your comfort level. You may progressively try more complex variants as your strength and flexibility improve.

9. Tranquillity and Meditation:

Incorporate mindfulness exercises and brief meditation sessions to create mindful moments.

To develop mental clarity and relaxation, this may be as easy as paying attention to your breath or utilizing applications that provide guided meditation.

10. Assess and Adjust:

After every session, set aside some time for introspection. Take note of your physical and mental well-being, any difficulties you face, and your progress. Make the appropriate adjustments to your practice.

11. Be patient and consistent:

Procedure: Form a consistent practice regimen. To enjoy the long-term advantages of yoga, consistency is essential.

Patience: Give your progress some time. Every yoga practice advances your wellbeing and personal development since it's a journey.

12. Seek Advice When Necessary:

Expert Advice: Should you be unsure about anything related to your health, think about speaking with a trained yoga teacher. Virtual meetings or online courses provide individualized instruction.

In conclusion, It is a powerful and rewarding undertaking to begin yoga at home. You may develop a meaningful and long-lasting practice that suits your unique requirements and preferences by clearing a space that is suitable to practicing mindfulness, using internet resources, making reasonable objectives, and giving it priority. Every yoga practitioner's path is different and offers not just physical advantages but also a deep examination of inner harmony and self-awareness.

Yoga Breath Awareness Techniques: An In-Depth Look at Mindful Breathing

A yoga journey is more than just physical poses; it's also an intentional investigation of the breath. Yoga's breath awareness practices link the body, mind, and spirit, acting as a transforming portal. We explore a variety of methods in this extensive book that promote mindfulness and aware breathing, enhancing and deepening your yoga practice.

1. Full Yogic Breath, or Diaphragmatic Breathing:

Method: Take a comfortable seat or lay down, making sure your spine is straight.
Put your hands on your abdomen and your chest, respectively.
Breathe deeply through your nose and feel your abdomen fill up completely.
As you fully and slowly release your breath via your nose, feel your abdomen constrict.

Maintain this regular breathing while highlighting the diaphragm's expansion.

Goal: Diaphragmatic breathing has a relaxing impact on the neurological system, expands lung capacity, and encourages relaxation. It serves as the cornerstone of mindful breathing.

2. The Victorious Breath, or Ujjayi Breath:

Method: Fill your lungs with a deep inhale via your nose.
-As you exhale through your nose, gently contract the back of your throat to produce a faint, audible sound.
-Continue to gently tighten while inhaling and exhaling.
-Breathing should be steady, effortless, and just barely audible.

Goal: Ujjayi breath improves focus, increases body temperature, and lends a contemplative aspect to the exercise. Because of its calming sound, it's often referred to as "ocean breath.".

3. Alternate Nostril Breathing, or Nadi Shodhana:

Method: Take a comfortable seat and maintain a straight back.
-Close your right nostril with your thumb, then take a deep breath in through your left.
-Using the right ring finger, shut the left nostril, let go of the right nostril, and release the breath.
-Breathe in via your right nostril, shut it, and then release the air through your left.
-Continue in this cycle, being cautious and slow.

Goal: Nadi Shodhana increases mental clarity, soothes the nervous system, and balances the two hemispheres of the brain. It's a really effective technique for balance and centering.

4. Square Breathing, or Box Breathing:

Technique: Breathe in for four counts.
-Hold your breath for four counts.
-Let go for four counts.
-Hold the breath for an additional four counts.
-Continue in this manner, progressively raising the number if it seems right.

Goals: Box breathing creates a feeling of equilibrium in the breath, eases anxiety, and encourages relaxation. It's a simple yet effective method for achieving a sense of calm and concentration.

5. Bee Breath, or Bhramari Pranayama:

Method: Take a comfortable seat and shut your eyes.
-Take a deep breath in through your nose.
Release your breath gently and make a bee-like buzzing sound.
-Throughout the exhale, keep your pitch constant and concentrate on the vibration in your brain.
- Carry out many rounds.

The goal of Bhramari pranayama is to create calmness, reduce tension, and calm the nervous system. The exercise takes on a new level as the humming quality activates the voice chords.

6. The "Skull Shining Breath," or Kapalabhati:

Method: Sit with your back straight.
-Inhale deeply, then expel air with power by tightening your abdominal muscles.
-Let the inhalation happen naturally.
-Start out slowly and pick up the pace over time.
-Complete rounds, then resume your regular breathing.

The purpose of kapalbhati is to stimulate the body, clear the respiratory system, and improve mental clarity and attention. It's a vigorous activity that enlivens the whole person.

In conclusion, breath awareness is the central concept that ties all the many aspects of yoga together; it is not just one of them. The variety of methods provided by these techniques enables practitioners to delve into the nuances of the breath. You may further strengthen the physical advantages of yoga and go on a journey towards inner balance, awareness and deep self-discovery by including these practices in your regimen. Let the breath be your guide as you go through these methods, incorporating awareness and tranquillity into all facets of your yoga practice.

A Comprehensive Guide to Breathing Techniques That Work for Cyclists and Runners

For runners and cyclists, breathing correctly is essential to achieving peak performance and endurance. Breathing strategies may be adjusted to meet the unique needs of various activities, which can result in increased oxygenation, less tiredness, and better general health. Let's take a closer look at a wide range of efficient breathing methods for bikers and runners.

1. Belly breathing, or diaphragmatic breathing:

Method: Breathe deeply through your nose, letting your belly swell to its maximum capacity.
Completely release the breath via your lips while tensing your abdominals.

Advantages: Involves the diaphragm for effective breathing.
increases oxygen intake and lung capacity.

Use: To build a solid basis for effective breathing, use diaphragmatic breathing throughout warm-ups and cool-downs.

2. Running Cadence Breathing:

Technique: Align your breath with your running cadence by taking one breath for every step and letting it out after the same number of strides.

Advantages: Breathe in time with your running to maintain a steady pace.

optimizes energy use and lowers the possibility of side stitches.

Applications: For increased endurance and effectiveness, use cadence breathing during training runs and competitions.

3. Cyclists' Nasal Breathing:

Method: While riding, inhale and exhale through your nose.

Advantages: Reduces respiratory system irritation by filtering and humidifying the air.
Controls airflow, which lowers the possibility of dehydration on long rides.

Use: Include nasal breathing in low-intensity rides to improve nasal breathing capacity and encourage effective respiration.

4. Endurance Box Breathing:

Method: Breathe in, hold it, release it, and then hold it again for the same number of counts (four seconds, for example).

Advantages: Improves lung capacity and respiratory control.

- Encourages relaxation and attention, which are essential for surviving difficult parts.

Use: - Include box breathing to help you stay calm and get the most oxygen throughout hard stretches or intervals.

5. Mindfulness with Breath:
Method: - Take a comfortable seat and concentrate on your breathing.
 - Pay attention to the breathing's natural rhythm.
 - Increase the length of the breaths you take in and out gradually.

Advantages: - Developing mindfulness and awareness of breathing patterns

- Assisting in stress reduction and mental clarity.

Use: - Include breath awareness meditation in your recovery regimen for general well-being or on days when you take a break.

6. Breathing Dynamically for Intervals:
Method: During the exercise phase, take a deep breath; during the recovery phase, release the breath quickly.

Advantages: align breathing at different intensities for interval exercise.
optimizes the amount of oxygen used during vigorous activity.

Use: To maximize energy distribution and recuperation during interval training, use dynamic breathing strategies.

7. Breath Pacing for Extended Exertions:

Technique: Create a regular breathing pattern by inhaling for three counts and exhaling for three counts.

Advantages: It keeps long-distance runs or rides moving at a steady, regulated pace.
reduces the possibility of exhaustion and dyspnea.
Use: To promote a focused and effective effort

during prolonged training sessions or races, use breath pacing.

8. Nadi Shodhana, or Alternate Nostril Breathing:
Method: Take a comfortable seat, shut one nostril, and breathe in through the other.
Exhale, open the other nostril, and close the one you just breathed.
Continue, switching up your nose.

Advantages: Reduces stress and balances energy pathways.
improves attention and concentration.

Use: Use alternating nostril breathing as a pre-race relaxing method or during the cool-down.

Conclusion, runners and cyclists may significantly improve their performance, endurance, and respiratory health by incorporating these various breathing strategies into their training regimens. Try these methods at various stages of your training cycle, and adjust your strategy to suit your preferences and the particular requirements of your sport. Breath control can be optimized through mindful application and consistent practice, which will promote a harmonious connection between movement and breath.

CHAPTER 5

RUNNERS' YOGA POSES

Runners may increase their flexibility, improve their circulation, and lower their chance of injury by doing a yoga warm-up before their run. This is an extensive regimen:

A Twisted High Lunge:

Hold for 15 to 30 seconds while twisting your body to face your front leg, starting from a lunge stance and bringing your hands to your heart. Carry out the same action on the other side.

Stretch on the side:

Place your feet hip-width apart, lift one arm above, and sag slightly to the other side. After 15 to 30 seconds of holding, swap sides.

Flowing Lunges:

Make a lunge step forward and then back to the starting position. To improve blood flow to the legs, repeat on the opposite leg for ten to fifteen repetitions.

Butterfly Extension:

Sit with your knees bent outward and the soles of your feet together. Holding onto your feet, gently expand your hips by flapping your knees up and down.

Forward Bend While Seated:

Lean back on your toes while sitting with your legs spread wide. To lengthen your hamstrings and lower back, hold for 15 to 30 seconds.

Position of the Pigeon:

Extend the second leg behind you while bringing one knee from a plank posture towards the wrist on the same side. After 15 to 30 seconds of holding, swap sides.

Stretch your quads while standing:

Place your foot near your buttocks while standing on one leg and bending the other knee. After 15 to 30 seconds of holding, swap legs.

Wind-Releasing Position:

Grasp your knee with both hands as you pull it close to your chest while lying on your back. After 15 to 30 seconds of holding, swap legs.

The Child's Position:

Reach your arms forward while kneeling on the mat and sitting back on your heels. To extend your shoulders and back, hold for thirty seconds.

Adaptive Arm Circles:

Make tiny circular movements with your arms out to the sides, progressively expanding the size of the circles. After fifteen seconds, change course.

Stretching the hamstrings:

With the sole of one foot pressed on the inner thigh and one leg extended, take a seat. Stretch out your leg and grasp its toes for a duration of 15 to 30 seconds. Alternate your legs.

Eagle Arms:

Bend your elbows, bring your palms together, and cross one arm over the other. Feel the upper back and shoulders expand as you raise your elbows to shoulder height.

Side leg lifts while standing:

One leg should be raised and then lowered as you stand with your hands on your hips. To engage the hip muscles, do 10 to 15 repetitions on each leg.

Mountain Position:

Reach your arms aloft and take a tall stance with your feet together. Before going for a run, take a 30-second break to concentrate on your breathing and centering yourself.

Last Stretch (Savasana):

For a few seconds, shut your eyes, lie on your back, and fully relax your body. As you prepare your thoughts for the impending run, concentrate on taking deep breaths.

In order to target different muscle groups and increase general flexibility and mobility for runners, this expanded practice includes extra stretches and dynamic exercises. Depending on your comfort level and time limits, change the length of each stretch.

- **Yoga Stretching Exercises:**

For runners, stretching using yoga poses before a run may help increase muscular strength, decrease the chance of injury, and improve flexibility. An in-depth tutorial on adding yoga stretches to your pre-run practice can be found here:

1. Uttanasana, or the Standing Forward Fold:

   In addition to stretching the hamstrings, this position decompresses the spine and improves alignment and posture. This is a great method to work your whole posterior chain, from your upper back to your calves.

2. Adho Mukha Svanasana, or Downward-Facing Dog:

   - Downward-facing dog not only stretches the shoulders, hamstrings, and calves, but it also tones the arms and legs. Stretching the whole body, it promotes spinal lengthening, which opens up the body and improves circulation.

3. Third Lunge (Anjaneyasana):

This lunge variant targets the hip flexors and quadriceps without overstretching the knee joint since the back knee remains on the ground. Because it replicates the motion of the running stride, it is very advantageous for runners.

4. Pose of the Seated Forward Bend (Paschimottanasana):

This position offers an intense stretch to the whole back, from the heels to the top of the head, as you bend forward. Prior to a run, it also helps to quiet the mind and promote mental concentration by stimulating the gastrointestinal organs and assisting in digestion.

5. Pigeon position (Eka Pada Rajakapotasana): -

Stretching the piriformis and hip flexors helps release stiffness in the hips, which makes this hip-opening position crucial for runners. Additionally, it may help to improve pelvic range of motion and relieve lower back stress.

6. Intense Leg Swings:

The dynamic leg swings provide mobility to the exercise, improving range of motion and flexibility. They prepare the muscles for the dynamic nature of running by targeting the hip joint particularly and warming them up in a useful way.

7. Chakravakasana also known as the Cat-Cow Stretch:

Cat and cow stretches are rhythmic and stimulate the core muscles in addition to warming the spine. It's a great method to increase spine flexibility and encourage fluidity in motion, both of which are essential for effective running.

8. Legs Up the Wall Pose (Viparita Karani):

This healing inversion promotes venous blood flow from the lower body back to the heart in addition to being a fantastic method to decompress the legs. Before your run, it may help you feel more rested and less fatigued in your legs by reducing swelling.

Not only can these yoga stretches help your body get ready for the physical demands of running, but they also help you develop body awareness and mindfulness. Maintaining consistency is essential, and stretching may increase performance by progressively lengthening each stretch. Always put emphasis on good form, pay attention to your body, and adjust postures to fit your unique requirements and capabilities.

CHAPTER 6

YOGA POSES FOR CYCLISTS

- **PRE-RIDE STRETCHING ROUTINE**

For cyclists to maximize performance, reduce risk of injury, and increase flexibility, a pre-ride stretching regimen is essential. Start with dynamic stretches to improve muscular suppleness by progressively raising heart rate and blood flow. Use arm circles, torso twists, and leg swings to work your primary muscle groups.

Target the quadriceps, hamstrings, and hip flexors by concentrating on the lower body with lunges and mild hamstring stretches. Work your way up to more specialized movements like knee hugs to engage your hip and gluteal muscles. Add ankle circles to enhance joint flexibility.

Shift to static stretches, holding each pose for 15–30 seconds to increase range of motion and lengthen muscles. Focus on the lower back, quadriceps, and calves. To ease stress, gently extend your neck.

Exercises like plank variants that emphasize core stability may help maintain posture and lessen the likelihood of lower back pain during rides. Remember to extend your upper body as well. To release tension from grasping the handlebars, do wrist rotations and shoulder stretches.

It's important to maintain consistency and modify the regimen as needed. In addition to preparing the body for the demands of cycling, a comprehensive pre-ride stretching regimen also helps ensure a fun and injury-free riding exexperience.

-Yoga Stretches For Cyclists Before Riding

Cycling puts special demands on the muscles and joints with its repetitive pedal strokes and prolonged body postures. Bicyclists may benefit from a customized series of yoga stretches that target the regions prone to tension and imbalances in order to guarantee a seamless and injury-free ride. Now let's explore these unique stretches further, which are intended to enhance a cyclist's pre-ride routine.

1. The Eagle Pose for Cyclists, or Garudasana for Cyclists:

Repetitive lateral motions used in cycling work the outer thighs and hips. The Eagle Pose for Cyclists is designed to specifically target these regions. Cycling may help to increase flexibility in the outer hip area by crossing one thigh over the other and bending the legs. This stretch improves stability during lateral bike motions in addition to relieving stress.

2. Ardha Matsyendrasana Variation of the Chainring Twist:

Cycling's rotating motion strains the core and lower back. A version of Ardha Matsyendrasana that targets this need for spinal flexibility is the Chainring Twist. During cycling, bikers spin their torsos repeatedly, which works the muscles in their lower back and core. Including this exercise in your pre-ride routine helps to avoid the soreness and stiffness that come with rotating motions.

3. Pedal Pusher's Pose (An Alternate Version of Suppa Virasana)

A common cause of tension for cyclists, the IT band needs careful attention. A version of Supta Virasana, the Pedal Pusher's Pose involves extending one leg to the side and reaching to the other side. This specific stretch helps to relieve tension in the outer thigh and hips, which improves pedal stroke and lowers the chance of problems with the IT band.

4. Handlebar Hinge (Uttanasana variation):

The forward-leaning posture of the bike causes pain in the shoulders and upper back for cyclists. This is addressed in the Handlebar Hinge, a version of Uttanasana that involves folding forward and clasping hands behind the back. This stretch helps to improve posture and general comfort during rides by relieving pressure on the shoulders and upper back.

5. Cogs and Cranks (Malasana Version):

Flexibility in the groin and hips is necessary for an effective pedal stroke. A variant of Malasana called Cranks & Cogs concentrates on these regions. The squatting posture works the groin and hip joint, increasing the flexibility needed for a smooth pedal stroke. Consistently doing this stretch improves the efficiency of your pedaling action.

6. Spoke Stretch (Janu Sirsasana parivrtta):

The Spoke Stretch is a great all-around stretch that works on both hip opening and spine rotation. The hip joint and spine are more flexible in cyclists, which helps them adjust to the dynamic nature of riding. This stretch improves your body's general range of motion, making your ride more comfortable and adaptable.

7. Handlebar Forward Fold (Shoulder Opener with Uttanasana):

Anxiety in the upper back and shoulders might make it difficult for a cyclist to ride. This problem is addressed by the Handlebar Forward Fold with a shoulder opening. Bicyclists may improve overall comfort and lower their chance of experiencing pain on longer rides by opening their shoulders wide during the forward fold.

8. Saddle Stretch (A Variation of Baddha Konasana):

- Sit with your feet flat on the ground and arrange your legs in a diamond formation.

- Feel the stretch in your inner thighs and groin as you gently push your knees toward the floor.

- This stretch works on the muscles that might become tense while riding a bike for an extended period of time.

9. Extension of the Aeroplane (Virabhadrasana III Variation):

- Place your feet hip-width apart, take a step back with your right foot, and bend your hips to stretch your arms forward.

- This version of Virabhadrasana III mimics the aerodynamic stance on the bike by stretching the back and engaging the core.

10. Peloton Plank (Phalakasana Variation):

- While maintaining a plank posture, engage your core by bringing your right knee to your right elbow.

- Go back to the plank and alternate sides.

- This vigorous exercise develops the muscles needed for stability during riding and heats the core.

11. Wheel Pose (Known as Urdhva Dhanurasana):

- Place your feet hip-width apart, bend your knees, and lie on your back.

- Raise your hips toward the ceiling by applying pressure with your hands and feet.

- This backbend counteracts the forward-leaning position on the bike by opening the chest and using the whole back.

12. Cadence Cobra (Bhujangasana variation):

- While lying prone, raise your chest and stretch your arms outward.

- Using your arms to simulate cycling, concentrate on deliberate, rhythmic motions.

- This stretch works the shoulders, lower back, and core, getting them ready for the cadence of cycling.

13. Getting Ready for the Upavistha Konasana (Groin Stretch):

- Take a seat with your legs wide apart. Bend forward at the hips.

- This stretch works the groin and inner thighs, increasing the flexibility needed for different cycling motions, particularly ascents.

14. Handlebar Hug (Adaptation of Child's Pose):

- Begin in child's pose and extend your arms in front of you.

- As if you were clutching fictitious handlebars, rotate your palms outward and bring your hands closer together.

- This stretch prepares riders for the handlebar grip by concentrating on the shoulders and upper back.

Finally, by including these extra yoga stretches in a rider's regimen, pre-ride preparation may be approached more thoroughly. Every stretch targets distinct muscle groups and gait patterns, guaranteeing a comprehensive warm-up for the body. Keep in mind to attentively execute these stretches, observing your body's reaction and customizing the exercise regimen to suit your demands. Maintaining a regular routine of these exercises will not only help to improve muscular imbalances and flexibility, but it will also strengthen the mind-body connection and make riding more pleasurable and satisfying.

Beyond just physical preparation, there are other benefits to using these unusual yoga poses in a pre-ride regimen. These stretches, with their deliberate breathing and targeted motions, help promote mental clarity, concentration, and an attentive attitude toward the ride. In addition to experiencing less muscular imbalances and more flexibility, cyclists also gain from a better overall riding experience. To fully use these stretches and make sure cyclists are prepared to face the road ahead with resilience and agility, it is essential to include them into the pre-ride routine consistently.

- **Warm-up Cycling Poses Before Yoga**

Cycling enthusiasts know how important it is to warm up properly before heading out on the road, and many have discovered that adding yoga poses improves both their general health and performance. Let's examine each component of the pre-yoga cycling warm-up in more detail, focusing on certain exercises and the advantages they provide riders.

1. Static Expansion:

Dynamic stretching is essential for preparing the body for exercise before cycling. Both backward and forward leg swings work the hip flexors and quads. The lubricating effects of hip and shoulder circles assist the joints get ready for the repeated actions of cycling.

2. Graces du Sun:

Sun Salutations are a basic yoga sequence that consist of a series of positions that flow into each other smoothly. Riders like the comprehensive advantages as the drill works every muscle in the body. In order to create a well-rounded warm-up, forward bends work the hamstrings while upward and downward dog postures strengthen and stretch the shoulders and back.

3. Activation of Core:

For cyclists, the core is their powerhouse, and being engaged with it is essential to maintaining bike stability. Plank variants like the side plank and high plank efficiently engage the core muscles. By forcing cyclists to use their abdominal muscles, the boat stance helps them improve their posture and endurance when riding.

4. Hip Starters:

Because they ride in a sitting posture, cyclists often report having stiff hips. The hip flexors are extensively stretched in the pigeon posture, which involves extending one leg behind and folding the other in front. Stretches like butterfly posture and lizard pose also work the hips, increasing hip flexibility and reducing soreness while riding.

5. Equilibrium Positions:

It is impossible to emphasize how crucial balance is for cyclists navigating a variety of terrains. One foot is placed on the inside thigh of the other leg in tree posture, which strengthens the lower body and tests balance. Eagle posture and Warrior III further increase stability, which improves control when riding a bike.

6. Inhalation Techniques:

Incorporate awareness into your warm-up routine with pranayama exercises. Cycling enthusiasts may develop a stable breathing technique by concentrating on diaphragmatic expansion via deep belly breathing. Breathing through one nostril at a time, or alternate nostril breathing, helps to soothe the nervous system and promotes a calm and concentrated state of mind prior to the ride.

7. Neural Flexibility:

Because of the forward-leaning posture on the bike, cyclists often get lower back stiffness. Cat-cow exercises increase lumbar flexibility by having the spine alternate between rounding and arching. In order to release tension and prime the spine for the dynamic action of cycling, seated twists gently rotate the spine.

8. Strengthening of Legs:

Even while cycling is largely a lower body exercise, it is still beneficial to strengthen your legs further. With their deep lunges, warrior postures work the glutes and quads. A more forceful pedal stroke may be achieved by engaging in chair stance, which tests the thighs and strengthens the core.

9. Shoulder and Neck Release:

During a ride, tension in the shoulders and neck might make a cyclist less comfortable. Releasing tension with gentle neck stretches, shoulder rolls, and neck rotations helps you relax and avoid pain on long rides.

10. Conscientious Visualization:

Bicyclists benefit from mental preparation in addition to physical preparation. Visualizing a successful and joyful ride while paying attention to the feelings, sights, and sounds is known as mindful or conscientious visualization. Bicyclists may approach their journeys with a more positive attitude and more attention thanks to this mental practice.

Cyclists may enjoy a thorough preparation that not only improves physical preparedness but also helps to mental resilience and a more satisfying riding experience by including these specific pre-yoga cycling warm-up activities into their practice.

- **POSITS FOR POST-RIDE RECOVERY**

Post-ride recovery postures are an essential part of a cyclist's overall approach to health and wellness because they provide a crucial link between the physical strain of a ride and the recuperation required for optimum physical health. These poses provide a therapeutic contrast to the repeated movements and muscular activation inherent in pedalling, and are specifically designed to meet the demands that cycling exerts on the body.

With its emphasis on lower body muscles and prolonged postures, cycling may eventually cause weariness, imbalances, and tense muscles. In order to offset these effects, post-ride recovery postures work to promote flexibility, release tension, and aid in the body's healing processes.

Targeting the main muscle groups used while cycling with mild stretches is an essential part of post-ride rehabilitation. The purpose of these stretches is to increase range of motion, increase flexibility, and relieve built-up tension. In this context, poses like forward folds, hip openers, and mild spinal twists are very helpful. They promote blood flow to tired muscles, assisting in the elimination of waste products from metabolism and streamlining the supply of vital nutrients needed for recuperation.

Moreover, deep breathing and relaxation are often included in post-ride recovery postures. During long rides, cyclists may feel more physically and mentally stressed. In these situations, restorative postures that promote mindful breathing might be beneficial. Breathing deeply and deliberately may assist trigger the parasympathetic nervous system, which in turn helps the body transition from an alert, energetic state to a more relaxed, resting one.

Bicyclists may also take advantage of these recovery poses to treat any areas of pain or imbalance that may have developed throughout the ride. Targeted postures may provide relief from any tightness in the body, including lower back, shoulder, and leg pain, as well as help avoid the build-up of tension and pressure that may eventually result in injury.

In summary, post-ride recovery postures go beyond the physical components of muscle regeneration; they extend to mental and emotional well-being. Cycling is not merely a physical sport; it stimulates the mind and body in conjunction. Incorporating positions that encourage relaxation and mental clarity may be as crucial as the physical advantages. One such example is the corpse position, or savasana, when cyclists may lay down in silence and let their body and mind fully absorb the healing effects of the ride and the recovery postures that follow.

Some Of The Yoga Poses After Cycling To Rehabilate Are:

1. Balasana (Child Pose):

Start by sitting back on your heels, stretching your arms forward so that your hands are resting on the floor, and kneeling on the mat. Reduce tension in your thighs, hips, and lower back as you sink into this healing position. To encourage a little stretch along the spine, place your forehead on the mat. Breathe deeply, opening up the rib cage. As you release each breath, release yourself into the posture, allowing your hips to progressively drop into your heels.

2. Viparita Karani's "Legs Up the Wall":

Place yourself next to a wall and lay on your back with your legs pressed up against the wall for this reviving inversion. To provide a pleasant and long-lasting stretch, use a folded blanket or bolster to support your lower back. This position helps the legs release stored lactic acid, which eases tightness in the muscles. Let's get rid of any remaining stress while you stay in this posture and enjoy the relaxing benefits on the neurological system.

3. Sarvangasana (Supported Shoulderstand):

As you elevate your legs toward the ceiling while lying on your back, use your hands to support your lower back. This inversion helps to extend the spine gently, improve circulation, and lessen leg edema. For extra support, place a folded blanket beneath your shoulders.

4. Bending Forward While Seated (Paschimottanasana):

Stretch your legs out in front of you while sitting, then reach for your toes with a hip-hinging motion. This forward bend helps to relieve tension in the lower back and hamstrings at the same time. For maximum stretch, maintain a straight spine. If you find it difficult to become flexible, you may progressively deepen the position by wrapping a strap over your feet. Allow your breathing to lead you into a relaxed, surrendered state.

5. Aloha Pose / Garland Pose:

Put your heels on the ground and your feet close together to form a squat. Press your legs outward with your elbows as you bring your hands together at your heart. Malasana helps with post-ride recuperation by extending the lower back, groin, and ankles.

6.Bridge Pose with Support:**

Rest on your back, knees bent, and place your feet hip-width apart. Raise your hips and place a support or block under your sacrum for stability. This version of Bridge Pose expands the chest and releases tension in the lower back. As you maintain the posture, concentrate on opening up the chest and feeling grounded in your hips to promote relaxation and healing.

7. Supta Matsyendrasana, (Supine Twist):

On your back, with your other shoulder still firmly planted, slowly lift one knee up to your chest and move it across your torso. This spherical stance increases general mobility and offers a mild relaxation for the spine. Breathe in a way that makes the rotation easier, opening up the torso and promoting space.

8. Pose for Needle Threading:

Lower the shoulder to the mat by sliding one arm beneath the other from a tabletop posture. The upper back and shoulders, which are often strained during riding, are the focus of this position. Feel the muscles in your upper back and shoulder gently relax as you thread the needle, encouraging a feeling of softness and relaxation.

9. Pose of the Butterfly (Baddha Konasana):

Sit like a butterfly with your knees bent outward and the soles of your feet together. Make rhythmic motions with your knees while you gently flap them. By opening the hips and inner thighs, this position relieves tension that builds up during riding. Letting go of any remaining tension and embracing the fluttering movement can help the hips expand and relax gradually.

10. Default Position (Savasana):

Lie on your back with your legs outstretched and your arms at your sides to complete your post-cycling yoga pose. Shut your eyes and focus on your breathing. Savasana promotes relaxation and mental clarity by allowing your body to absorb the benefits of the practice. Release any residual tension while you hold this posture, allowing a profound sensation of healing and tranquillity to surround you. Take at least five to ten minutes to remain in Savasana so that your body and mind may thoroughly absorb the restorative benefits of your practice.

11. Supported Fish Pose (A Modification of Matsyasana):

Sit with your mid-back supported by a block or bolster, then lean back over it. By gently arching the back, you may counterbalance the forward-leaning posture that comes with riding a bike. To improve the stretch and relieve tension in the upper body, concentrate on taking deep breaths.

12. Bend Forward While Standing (Uttanasana):

Place your feet hip-width apart, bend at the hips, and extend your reach to the ground. The lower back, calves, and hamstrings are all stretched in uttanasana. Encouraging a mild release in the spine and fostering relaxation, let the upper body swing freely.

13. Pose of the Lizard (Utthan Pristhasana):

Lower your forearms to the floor and place one foot on the outside edge of the mat while in a lunge stance. Stretching the hips, groin, and hamstrings profoundly is what Lizard Pose does. Accept the slow expansion of the hips and let the breath lead you into a deeper stretch.

14. (Garudasana Arms) Eagle Arms:

Raise your arms in front of you, placing your palms together and crossing one over the other. Raise your elbows while maintaining a relaxed shoulder posture. This position releases stress and improves upper body flexibility by focusing on the shoulders and upper back.

15. Hand-to-Big-Toe Pose in Reclining (Supta Padangusthasana):

Stretch one leg toward the ceiling while laying on your back and support it with your hand by the big toe. If necessary, use a strap to keep the stretch comfortable. The hamstrings and calves, which are often strained during riding, are the focus of this position. Accept the leg's extension and pay attention to how the rear of the leg is gently opening. Strike a balance between effort and relaxation in the stretch, and let the breath lead the way.

Including these intricate and subtle yoga positions into your post-riding regimen provides a multidimensional strategy for physical recuperation. Every posture has a different emphasis and set of advantages, but all of them help cyclists feel better overall by increasing their flexibility, releasing tight muscles, and cultivating a deep feeling of calm. Adopt these strategies to improve your recuperation process and guarantee continued fun and efficiency in your riding pursuits.

YOGA ROUTINE TO COOL DOWN FOR CYCLISTS

For cyclists, a well-planned yoga cool-down sequence is crucial, as it offers a conscious shift from the intensity of riding to a relaxed, recuperative state. The goals of this program should be to promote mental clarity, increase flexibility, and release stress. Let's investigate a range of distinctive and useful yoga poses designed especially for bikers as cool-down exercises.

1. Bananasana (Banana Pose):

Stretch your arms above while maintaining a straight posture with your legs. Gently turn your hips to the side so that your body resembles a banana. This lateral stretch lengthens the intercostal muscles and fosters an open feeling by releasing tension along the sides of the torso.

2. Asana Maksikanagasana (Dragonfly Pose):

Place your legs wide apart and bend forward from the hips while sitting. This forward fold with broad legs stretches the groins, hamstrings, and inner thighs. Additionally, it offers a mild relaxation for the lower back, which is very comforting after a ride.

3. Gomukhasana (Cow Face Pose) Arms bent sideways:

Put your hands together behind your back and stack your right elbow over your left. Make a little bend to the right with your lean. This position provides relaxation for the lateral muscles and upper body while focusing on the shoulders, triceps, and side body.

4. Neck rotation in Sphinx Pose:

With your elbows under your shoulders and your chest up, lie on your stomach. Turn your head from side to side to include a neck rotation. While the neck rotates to relieve tension in the cervical spine, Sphinx Pose stretches the front of the body and activates the lower back.

5. Utthan Pristhasana or Lizard Pose:

Lower your forearms to the floor inside your front leg from a low lunge. This deep hip opener works the hamstrings, groin, and hip flexors. Moreover, it promotes gradual relaxation in the lower back, which is very advantageous for bikers.

6. Sitting Forward Bend with Wide Legs (Upavistha Konasana):

Place your legs wide apart and bend forward from the hips while sitting. The inner thighs and hamstrings are deeply stretched in this position. To assist with your forward fold and provide a pleasant release, use props like blocks or a bolster.

7. Pose of the Twisted Monkey (Parivrtta Malasana):

Grasp the mat with both hands while in a deep squat, then rotate your body to extend one arm upward. This posture releases tension in the spine and promotes hip flexibility by combining a deep hip opener with a spinal twist.

8. Leg lifts in supine butterfly pose (supta baddha konasana):

With your legs wide apart and the soles of your feet touching, lie on your back. Incorporate leg raises to activate the inner thighs and progressively fortify the abdominal muscles. The advantages of the traditional Butterfly Pose are amplified by this version.

9. Ardha Matsyendrasana (Half Lord of the Fishes Pose) with Side Bend:

Stretch one leg out in front of you while sitting, then lay your other foot over it. To extend the stretch further, twist in the direction of the bowed knee and add a side bend. This position provides a multi-faceted relief, working on the hips, side body, and spine.

10. Supported Reclining Bound Angle Pose (Supta Baddha Konasana) with Bolster:

Position a bolster under your spine for support while lying on your back with your legs apart and the soles of your feet together. This healing version of Bound Angle position encourages a little opening in the hips, which makes it the perfect position to end your cool-down.

11. The Uttana Shishosana, or puppy pose:

Place yourself on a tabletop and move your hips over your knees while you walk your hands forward. This posture extends the shoulders, lengthens the spine, and eases some of the tension in the lower back.

Include these modified yoga positions in your cool-down to provide a customized and comprehensive approach to recuperation after riding. As you go from the physical demands of cycling to a state of comfort and repair, keep your breathing steady the whole time to promote awareness and relaxation.

POSES FOR CORE STRENGTH AND BALANCE FOR CYCLISTS

Those who ride bikes often look for yoga positions that effectively strengthen their cores in order to improve their general stability and riding prowess. Maintaining good posture, enhancing balance, and effectively transmitting power during pedal strokes all depend on core strength.

In addition to increasing their leg strength and cardiovascular fitness, cyclists often aim to improve their performance by emphasizing core strength and balance. Better overall control, efficient energy transfer, and increased stability on the bike are all attributed to having a strong core and excellent balance. Let's explore in detail some particular yoga positions that work on both balance and core strength to provide riders a complete training program.

Let's explore a range of striking and effective yoga positions designed especially to help bikers develop their core muscles.

1. Boat Pose:

A basic yoga posture, boat pose works the whole core, including the deep stabilizing muscles and the rectus abdominis. In order to increase the intensity and target various regions of the core, cyclists may do variants such as dynamic boat stance, which involves rising and lowering the legs.

2. Vasisthasana, or Side Plank:

The side plank is a great exercise to work the lateral muscles and obliques. Cyclists use their whole core by raising their hips and keeping their body in a straight line from head to heels. Stability and rotational strength are also tested by variations such as inserting a needle into a side plank. This position works the core and encourages lateral mobility to maintain balance on the bike.

3. Dolphin Plank Position:

Dolphin posture, which combines aspects of downward dog and plank, is an energetic pose that tones the whole core. The activation of the stabilizing muscles and lower abdominals helps cyclists build a stronger core foundation.

4. Pose for Relieving the Wind (Pavanamuktasana):

Wind-relieving stance, while mostly associated with digestive benefits, works the core muscles as bikers bring one leg at a time toward the chest. This exercise helps alleviate tension in the lower back while focusing on the lower abs.

5. Holding a Hollow Body pose:

The hollow body hold is a gymnastics-inspired position in which the practitioner lies on their back, raises their legs and upper body off the floor, and forms a tiny "U" shape. The whole core, including the often underutilized lower abdominal muscles, is vigorously activated in this position.

6. Pose of the Crow (Bakasana):

Although crow pose seems to be an arm balance, lifting the legs off the ground demands strong core muscles. This stance helps cyclists gain general balance and core stability, which helps them handle the bike more precisely.

7. Plank with elbow to knee:

Adding a controlled element to the classic plank, riders may raise their knee to the opposing elbow. This exercise works the obliques and improves coordination, both of which are important for sustaining control across a variety of terrains.

8. Pose of a Fire Hydrant:

Fire hydrant posture is a great way to work on your outer thighs and hip abductors, but it is often ignored. By making these muscles stronger, you may avoid excessive side-to-side cycling movement and improve overall stability.

9. Trikonasana (Extended Triangle Pose):

Standing in extended triangle posture, you may stretch your legs and strengthen your core at the same time. Stretch one arm down to your shin or a block while extending the other arm upwards, keeping your legs wide apart.

A spin on the classic triangle stance, tests a rider's ability to maintain stability while turning and works the obliques. Enhancing rotational strength is necessary for smooth bike riding, and this stance does just that.

10. Adho Mukha Vrksasana, or handstand:

Even for skilled handstanders, maintaining balance when inverted takes a strong core engagement. Cyclists may progressively develop their strength and stability by practicing with a spotter or against a wall.

12. Vrksasana (Tree Pose):

A traditional yoga practice that tests equilibrium and strengthens the core is tree pose. Place the sole of your other foot on your inner thigh or calf while standing on one leg. While raising the arms aloft, try to keep your balance by focusing on anything. In addition to strengthening the core, this position enhances stability in a single-leg stance, which is akin to riding.

13. Virabhadrasana III (Warrior III):

Balance and core involvement are combined in the dynamic stance known as Warrior III. Hinge at the hips and stretch your arms forward while straightening one leg backwards while standing. The body becomes a T-shape, which engages the core and encourages a steady, streamlined posture.

14. Phalakasana, or Plank Pose:

A fundamental stance that helps develop core strength is plank pose. Start by placing your wrists below your shoulders in the push-up posture. Keep your body in a straight posture from head to heels and engage your core. In addition to targeting the obliques, variations like side plank aid in the development of a well-rounded core.

15. Ardha Chandrasana, or Half Moon Pose:

Balance and strength are combined in half moon pose. After doing Warrior II, transfer your weight onto one leg, elevate your rear leg parallel to the floor, and extend your front arm downward. In addition to strengthening general stability and attention, this position works at the core.

16. Tittibhasana, or Firefly Pose:

The advanced arm balance known as Firefly Pose works the core and calls for a keen sense of balance. Stretch your legs out from under you, raising them off the ground, while keeping your hands on the mat. Both stability and core strength are required for this stance.

17. Tolasana or Scale Pose:

Scale Pose is an arm balance that tests both balance and core strength at the same time. Stretch your legs out in a sitting position, put your hands on the mat next to your hips, and raise your legs off the floor. It takes a strong core to stay balanced in the raised posture in this pose. Strengthen your core to maintain balance in this raised posture, benefiting your cycling performance.

A cyclist's balance, core strength, and general stability on the bike may all be greatly improved by including these yoga positions into their training regimen. By strengthening the body's capacity to maintain stability during dynamic movements and treating core deficits, regular practice of these postures not only improves performance but also helps avoid injuries. These positions may be used into a cyclist's cross-training program to promote a holistic approach to physical health and riding ability.

The secret is to remain consistent, to use good technique, and to work your way up to more difficult versions as your core muscles become stronger.

Some Additional Yoga Poses and Techniques To Help Cyclists Achieve Better Balance

Improving one's balance is essential to riding a bike since it increases stability, which is particularly important while riding on difficult terrain. A cyclist's practice may be greatly enhanced by including a variety of yoga postures, which target various muscle groups and increase proprioception, so improving overall balance. Here, we'll explore distinctive and different yoga poses designed to improve cyclists' balance.

1. Half Moon Pose with Rotation (Parivrtta Ardha Chandrasana):

- Place your right foot forward to begin in Warrior I.

- Position the right hand inside the right foot, either on the ground or on a block.

Raise your left leg so that it is parallel to the floor and raise your left arm up toward the sky.

- Tighten your core and strike a balance between your outstretched leg and your supporting hand.

2. Ustrasana (Camel Pose):

- Place your knees hip-width apart on the mat.

- Put your hands on your lower back and tuck your toes beneath.

- Bend your back and extend your hands to your heels.

- To maintain balance, keep your hips over your knees and contract your core.

3. Vasisthasana (Side Plank):

- Take a plank stance to start.

- Place your weight on the outside of your right foot and right hand.

- Raise the left arm toward the heavens and place the left foot atop the right.

- Find balance in a side plank posture by using your core.

4. Anomalous Object (Camatkarasana):

- Make a downward dog start.

Raise your right leg, bending your knee and opening your hips.

- Turn your body such that your right foot is on the ground behind your left leg.

- Form an arch with your left arm by reaching it forward.

5. Malasana Garland Pose:

- Place your feet wider apart than your hip width apart.

- Drop to a squat, putting your body between your thighs.

- To maintain balance, place your hands together in the middle of your heart and squeeze your elbows on your inner thighs.

6. Parivrtta Utkatasana, or Revolved Chair Pose):

- Place your feet together in a chair pose to start.

- Rotate the body to one side while extending one elbow across the leg of the other person.

- Maintain balance by keeping your knees together and using your core.

7. Headstand (Salamba Sirsasana) Supported:

- Place your forearms on the mat to begin in Dolphin Pose.

- Move your feet closer to your face and raise your hips toward the ceiling.

Elevate one leg at a time until you are able to balance on your head's crown.

8. Halasana, or Plow Pose:

- While lying on your back, raise your legs upward and bring them toward the floor.

- Extend the legs for a deep stretch while using your hands to support your lower back.

To keep your balance and composure during this inversion, contract your core.

9. Navasana Boat Pose Variation:

Sit on the mat with your feet flat and your knees bent.

- Raise the feet off the floor and stretch the legs upward.

Slightly recline, maintaining your balance on the sitting bones, and extend your arms or place your hands behind your thighs.

Including these many yoga positions in a rider's practice provides a comprehensive method of improving balance. Every posture works on certain muscle groups, has unique stability issues, and enhances proprioception overall. Regular practice of these stances helps a rider feel more focused and confident when riding, as well as improving their ability to maneuver over challenging terrain.

CHAPTER 7

BREATHWORK FOR ENDURANCE

- **Pranayama Running Techniques:**

Yoga's pranayama, or breath control technique, provides helpful methods for runners who want to run more efficiently, build endurance, and practice mindfulness. A runner's regimen may benefit from using pranayama as it helps optimize oxygen intake, reduce tension, and foster mental concentration. Here, we look into certain pranayama methods designed for runners:

1. Diaphragmatic Breathing (Deep Belly Breathing):

The diaphragm is expanded during deep belly breathing to facilitate maximal air intake. Running enthusiasts may use this method by taking a deep breath with their nose, letting their belly swell, and then completely expelling through their mouth. This promotes effective oxygen exchange and lessens the likelihood of shallow breathing during running.

2. Sama Vritti (Equal Breathing):

Sama Vritti calls for holding in breaths for the same amount of time as they are exhaled. It is possible for runners to create a rhythmic pattern by matching their breath to their steps. During a run, this strategy improves overall respiratory efficiency, balance, and breath control.

3. Alternate Nostril Breathing (Nadi Shodhana):

A peaceful pranayama method called nadi shodhana helps to balance the left and right hemispheres of the brain. This method may be used by runners to concentrate their minds before a run or to decompress after one. Running fosters a feeling of equilibrium and tranquility by switching between nostrils during intake and exhale.

4. Kapalabhati (Breath of the Shining Skull):

In kapalabhati, one must exhale firmly and then inhale passively. Running enthusiasts may find this energetic pranayama practice useful as it improves lung capacity, circulation, and creates a sensation of invigoration. To prevent overdoing it, you must practise Kapalbhati carefully and gently at first.

5. Ocean Breath (Ujjayi Breathing):

Ujjayi breathing produces a gentle, ocean-like sound by inhaling and exhaling via the nose while slightly tightening the back of the throat. This method may improve awareness, assist runners maintain a consistent breathing pattern, and help them more skillfully control the intensity of their runs.

6. Bee Breath (Bhramari):

Bhramari is a peaceful pranayama practice where you exhale and make a humming noise. Bhramari is a technique that runners may use to lower tension, relax the nervous system, and improve mental clarity. This method is very helpful for unwinding and recuperating after a run.

7. Sitali (the Breath of Cooling):

Sitali is a cooling technique that requires breathing via pursed lips or a curled tongue. This particular pranayama method helps runners in hotter weather by lowering body temperature, increasing overall comfort, and regulating body temperature.

8. Three-Part Breath (Dirga Pranayama):

The lower abdomen, chest, and upper lungs are the three areas of the breath that are focused on in Dirga Pranayama. By encouraging complete oxygen exchange and assisting runners in learning to breathe more widely, this strategy improves lung capacity and respiratory efficiency as a whole.

A runner's training program must include pranayama practices that are consistently practiced and tailored to their own preferences. Throughout their training, runners may include these strategies into their warm-ups, cool-downs, and even steady-state runs to enhance their breathing patterns, control their energy levels, and promote mental clarity and concentration.

- **Breathwork During An Endurance Run**

Breathwork is essential for increasing running endurance because it promotes a mind-body connection, energy management, and optimal oxygen intake. A runner's ability to retain mental concentration and sustain exertion over longer distances may be greatly enhanced by using proper breathing methods. Let's take a closer look at the main components of breathwork for running endurance.

1. Breathing Diaphragmatically:

Belly breathing, also referred to as diaphragmatic breathing, is taking deep breaths via the nose, letting the diaphragm fall, and filling the lungs with air. By optimizing oxygen exchange, this approach gives the muscles a greater amount of oxygen to work with during running. Additionally, it lessens chest breathing that is shallow, which increases tiredness.

2. Breathing in rhythm:

For endurance, breathing must be synchronised with your running rhythm. A 3:3 or 2:2 pattern, in which you inhale for three steps and exhale for three, is found to be efficient by many runners. By keeping the muscles' supply of oxygen constant, this synchronisation lowers the accumulation of carbon dioxide and improves respiratory efficiency all around.

3. Breathing via the nose:

Prior to the air entering the lungs, nasal breathing cleans, humidifies, and helps control breathing. By slowing down breathing via the nose, one may encourage a more steady and regulated breathing rate. When running at a low to moderate intensity, nasal breathing is very helpful.

4. Awareness of Breath:

When you run, you may cultivate mindfulness by focusing on the rhythm, depth, and sensation of your breath. This awareness enables runners to recognize patterns of stress or holding their breath and make appropriate corrections. Additionally, mindful breathing helps the runner stay in the present, which promotes attention and focus.

5. Breathe Out Deeply:

A thorough exhale is just as vital to effective breathwork as a full inhalation. A complete exhale helps free up space for a new oxygen intake by releasing carbon dioxide and stale air. Some runners discover that during longer runs, concentrating on a longer exhale may soothe the nervous system and encourage relaxation.

6. Controlling Breath in Hills and Intervals:

During hills or intervals, you must modify your breathing pattern in order to maintain energy control. In order to keep up with the increased demand for oxygen on uphill parts, many runners start to breathe faster and shorter. On the other hand, during downhill sections, regulated and deeper breathing promotes recovery and lessens the likelihood of muscular weariness.

7. Gradual Breath Exercise:

Progressive breath training includes doing breath-focused exercises during non-running activities at progressively higher intensities and longer durations. This might include doing yoga, setting aside time for breathwork, or integrating breath awareness into regular tasks. The respiratory muscles get more conditioned with progressive exercise, increasing their running efficiency.

8. Breathing Techniques for Recovery:

It's important to concentrate on recovery breathing after a run. This is taking deep diaphragmatic breaths, slowing down breathing, and letting the heart rate progressively return to normal. During the recovery period, controlled breathing helps to promote general healing and lessen muscular discomfort.

9. Practice Breathing:

Running-specific breathwork routines, such box breathing and pursed lip breathing, might be helpful. In order to promote regulated exhalation, pursed lip breathing entails inhaling through the nose and exhaling via pursed lips. Breathing patterns may be regulated and the nervous system can be calmed via box breathing, which involves breathing in equal and controlled phases.

In conclusion, breathwork for running endurance is a complex strategy that includes a range of methods to maximize oxygen uptake, control energy, and improve concentration. Including these exercises in a runner's training regimen may help them run with more endurance, less tiredness, and greater enjoyment in the process.

CYCLISTS' PRANAYAMA TECHNIQUES

The ancient yogic discipline of pranayama, or regulated breathing, provides cyclists with a useful toolkit for improving both their physical and mental health. These methods go beyond traditional aerobic exercise and provide riders ways to increase oxygen intake, sharpen their attention, and reduce stress. Since breathing and movement go hand in hand with riding, pranayama is a suitable and approachable addition to every cyclist's training program.

1.Bee Breath, Bhramari:

Bhramari, also known as bee breath, is a peaceful pranayama practice in which you exhale while making a humming noise. This method may help cyclists de-stress and calm their nerves, which will clear their minds and allow them to ride more intently. Bhramari is very helpful for relaxing during breaks or after a ride.

2. Dirga Pranayama or Three-Part Breath:

The three-part breath, or dirga pranayama, places emphasis on filling the lower, middle, and upper lungs in that order. This thorough breathwork promotes complete oxygen exchange and improves lung capacity. To enhance their respiratory function, cyclists might use the three-part breath during warm-up or cool-down periods.

3. Ujjayi Inhalation:

Ujjayi breathing, sometimes called "ocean breath" because it sounds like ocean waves, is good for cyclists who want to increase their mental stamina and attention. To produce a calming sound, this method entails gently tightening the back of the neck during inhalation and exhalation. Ujjayi breathing helps improve focus, which makes it especially helpful on lengthy rides or in difficult terrain.

4. Kapalabhati (Breath of the Shining Skull):

The energizing pranayama practice of kapalabhati consists of quick, strong exhalations followed by quiet inhalations. Invigorating the body, stimulating the abdominal muscles, and aiding with mental clarity, this dynamic breathwork is beneficial for bikers. Adding Kapalabhati to your pre-ride practice helps arouse your body and get it ready for the strenuous physical demands of cycling.

5. Breathing from the deep belly:

The core of bicycle pranayama is deep belly breathing, or diaphragmatic breathing. Cycling may improve respiratory efficiency by increasing oxygen intake by intentionally contracting the diaphragm and expanding the lower lungs. By establishing a link between breath and movement, this fundamental technique promotes a more regulated and rhythmic cycling experience.

6. Inhaling via the box:

Box breathing promotes balance and control since it involves equal intervals of intake, breath retention, expiration, and another breath retention. This is a strategy that cyclists may use to control their breathing, reduce anxiety, and improve focus during different stages of their rides.

7. Nostril Breathing Alternative (Nadi Shodhana):

Alternate nostril breathing, or nadi shodhana, is a balancing pranayama method that balances and harmonizes the body's energy flow. This is a method that cyclists may employ before or after rides to help with nervous system calmness, attention improvement, and balance. It encourages a balanced distribution of energy throughout the body by requiring breathing and exhaling via different nostrils

8. Meditation on Breath Awareness:

Beyond particular methods, bikers may practice mindfulness via breath awareness meditation. This is paying attention to the breath's natural flow and not trying to change it. This meditation technique improves resilience, mental clarity, and general well-being, all of which contribute to a satisfying riding experience.

In conclusion, including pranayama methods into a cyclist's regimen provides a comprehensive strategy for both mental and physical preparation. By improving respiratory efficiency, fostering attention, or regulating stress, these strategies provide cyclists an effective toolkit to maximize their performance and develop a stronger connection between their breath and their bike.

- **Breathing Activities For Cycling Stamina**

Cycling enthusiasts who want to increase their endurance and stamina during rides must prioritize breathing exercises. In addition to guaranteeing a continuous flow of oxygen to the muscles, effective breathing aids cyclists in reducing tiredness and improving their overall performance. Let's take a closer look at a variety of breathing techniques designed especially to increase riding endurance.

1.Pursed-Lip Inhalation:

In order to practice pursed-lip breathing, inhale through the nose and gently exhale through the lips. By generating back pressure, this method keeps the bronchioles from collapsing and preserves airflow. Breathing with your lips pursed helps throughout the most difficult parts of a trip.

2. Ujjayi Inhalation:

The "ocean breath," or ujjayi breath, is inhaled via the nose and exhales somewhat into the back of the throat. Cyclists who use this audible breath may improve their attention, deepen their inhalations, and control their breathing rate. Ujjayi breath is very helpful during hard sprints or difficult uphill hikes.

3. Box Breathing:

Many athletes utilize a method called box breathing, which is inhaling, holding the breath, expelling, and holding again for the same number of counts.

Bicyclists, for instance, may inhale for four counts, hold for four, exhale for four, and hold for four. This technique helps to maintain a constant beat, lessen anxiety, and manage breathing.

4. Cadence Alignment:

Syncing respiration with bicycle cadence may improve productivity. It is possible for cyclists to coordinate their breathing with their pedal strokes, inhaling completely during one pedal revolution and expelling during the next. This synchronization encourages respiratory and cardiovascular activity to flow in unison.

5. Breathing via the nose:

Prior to the air reaching the lungs, breathing via the nose warms, humidifies, and filters the air. In addition to engaging the lower lungs and activating the diaphragm, nasal breathing facilitates a more effective gas exchange. To increase their respiratory efficiency, cyclists might practise nasal breathing during low-intensity rides.

6. Breathing Diaphragmatically:

In order to enhance air intake, diaphragmatic breathing also referred to as deep belly breathing involves contracting the diaphragm. This may be practiced by cyclists by taking a deep breath via their nose, letting their diaphragm drop, and then expelling completely through their mouth. This method helps you stay calm during the ride and encourages effective oxygen exchange.

7. Breathing in rhythm:

Developing a regular breathing pattern is essential for endurance. It is possible for cyclists to develop a pattern where they inhale for two counts and exhale for two counts. Breathing rhythmically aids in controlling prolonged periods of exertion and energy consumption.

8. Breathing from the belly as you descend:

Cycling at fast speeds or when descending might cause riders to hold their breath unintentionally. When descending, deep belly breathing keeps the muscles' oxygen supply intact and keeps tension from building.

9. Meditation on Breath Awareness:

Including breath awareness meditation in one's cycling regimen improves breathing awareness and mindfulness. During brief meditation sessions, bikers may reduce overall tension on their bodies by connecting with their breathing patterns and promoting calm via breath-focused awareness.

10. Breathing Techniques for Recovery:

Cycling enthusiasts might benefit from intentional recovery breathing after strenuous exertion. To help with the elimination of metabolic waste products and improve recuperation, this entails slowing down breathing, taking deeper breaths, and exhaling completely.

Performing these breathing techniques on a regular basis will help you become a much better cyclist. By incorporating them into both training sessions and real rides, riders may improve their breathing awareness, effort management, and road endurance in the end.

CHAPTER 8

CONSCIOUSNESS AND MENTAL STRENGTH

- **Yoga as a Stress Reduction Technique**

Stress has become a common companion for many people in the fast-paced and often demanding world of contemporary living. Yoga has become a well-recognized holistic discipline that balances the mind, body, and spirit, making it an effective tool for stress relief. This review will examine the many ways that yoga may help reduce stress, as well as the methods, advantages, and different types of yoga that can help one become more resilient and at ease.

Recognizing Stress and Its Impacts:

Stress may show up as physical or mental symptoms, depending on what's causing it work, relationships, or other outside influences. Persistent stress may cause a wide range of health problems, from sleep disorders and anxiety to more serious ailments like heart disease. As a comprehensive strategy that tackles the underlying causes of stress and enhances general well-being, yoga is becoming more popular among those who understand the necessity of effective stress management.

Yoga as a Body-Mind Exercise

Fundamentally, yoga is a mind-body practice that incorporates movement, breath, and awareness rather than just being a physical workout. Asanas (physical postures), pranayama (breath control), and meditation work in deep harmony to support people in navigating and reducing stress.

- **Meditation and yoga as stress relievers:**

With their comprehensive approach to addressing the mental, emotional, and physical elements of stress, yoga and meditation are effective strategies for relieving stress. The synergistic impact of the concentrated attention of meditation and the mindful movement of yoga promotes calmness and relaxation. Let's examine the methods used in yoga and meditation to effectively reduce stress.

Using Yoga to Reduce Stress:

1. Soft Pose Asanas:

Physical stress may be released with the use of gentle yoga positions like cat-cow, legs-up-the-wall, and child's pose. In order to encourage a feeling of comfort in the body, these postures concentrate on opening and extending the places where tension tends to build up.

2. Pranayama Deep Breathing:

The foundation of yoga's approach to stress reduction is breath awareness. By triggering the body's relaxation response, methods such as diaphragmatic breathing and ujjayi breath (ocean breath) assist soothe the nervous system and lessen the physiological consequences of stress.

3. Nidra Yoga:

Yoga nidra is a guided meditation that creates a state of conscious relaxation; it is often referred to as "yogic sleep." In order to foster a profound feeling of peace and renewal, practitioners are led through many phases of relaxation.

4. Yoga for Regeneration:

This kind of yoga calls on holding passive postures with supports for lengthy periods of time. Deep relaxation is facilitated by restorative yoga, which helps the body let go of tension and stress. Particularly helpful poses are reclining bound angle stance and supported savasana.

5. Vinyasa Mindful Movement:

In addition to strengthening and extending the muscles, vinyasa yoga promotes meditation by having practitioners go through a series of postures with conscious breath synchronization. The flow of rhythm calms the mind and directs attention within.

Stress-Reduction Through Meditation:

1. Meditation with mindfulness:

Being mindful entails focusing on the here and now without passing judgment. You may practice this kind of meditation by paying attention to your breath, your body's sensations, or you can do it by monitoring your thoughts and emotions objectively. Stress reactivity is decreased by mindfulness, which develops a non-reactive awareness.

2. Metta's Loving-Kindness Meditation

Sending loving and compassionate thoughts to oneself and others is the practice of Metta meditation. By fostering a pleasant emotional state and strengthening a feeling of connectivity, this practice mitigates the detrimental consequences of stress.

3. Meditation in Transcendental:

In Transcendental Meditation (TM), a mantra is quietly repeated twice a day for fifteen to twenty minutes. By lowering tension and fostering a profound feeling of calm, this approach seeks to attain a state of peaceful awareness.

4. Meditation using Body Scan:

By focusing attention on various body areas during a body scan meditation, tension is gradually released and relaxation is encouraged. This mindfulness exercise is beneficial for fostering a mind-body connection and easing the physical pain brought on by stress.

5. Guided Visualization Exercise:

Using guided imagery, one may visualize serene and tranquil settings. This kind of meditation helps people decompress and become more mentally clear by taking them to a stress-free mental place.

Strategies to Improve Outcomes:

1. Coherence:

The secret is to practice often. The efficacy of yoga and meditation increases with time as a regular practice is established. Significant stress-relieving effects may be obtained from even brief daily sessions.

2. Awareness of Mind:

People may manage their stress in real time by incorporating mindfulness into their everyday activities as well as their formal practice. Eating, walking, and working mindfully all help one become more grounded and in the moment.

3. Flexibility:

A more customized and pleasurable experience is ensured by procedures that are tailored to individual tastes and demands. People might discover what kind of yoga and meditation most appeals to them by experimenting with different kinds.

4. Psycho-Somatic Link:

The mind-body connection is strengthened by placing emphasis on the integration of the mind and body during practice. Resilience to stress is cultivated by the nonjudgmental acknowledgment of thoughts, feelings, and sensations.

People may use yoga and meditation to effectively relieve stress by combining these practices into a comprehensive strategy. The combination of yoga postures and meditation, whether used for physical release or to develop mental clarity, provides a holistic and long-lasting strategy for stress management in the contemporary environment.

- **Mindfulness Exercises Among Cyclists and Runners:**

Running and cycling mindfulness techniques focus on developing an acute awareness of the present moment while engaging in physical exercise, encouraging a harmonious relationship between the mind and body. These behaviours improve general well-being in addition to performance. Let's discuss the many facets of mindfulness for cyclists and runners, how to incorporate these practices into training, and the possible advantages they may have for different bodily systems.

Conscious Inhalation:

Conscious breathing is one of the cornerstones of mindfulness. During activity, it might be beneficial for bikers and runners to be aware of their breathing. By concentrating on taking deep, regular breaths, one may control their intake of oxygen, which enhances their endurance and lessens their impact on the heart.

Meditation with a Body Scan:

Body scan meditations are useful for bikers and runners during cool-downs or stretching exercises. This is focusing on various bodily areas, identifying any tension or pain, and letting it go mindfully. By focusing on areas of tension, this technique improves body awareness and helps avoid injuries.

Being Aware While Cycling and Running:

One of the main components of mindfulness is giving the task at hand your whole attention. Enjoying the sensation of the earth under your feet or the breeze on your face when riding is enhanced when you are totally present in the moment. This increased awareness also aids in performance enhancement, form improvement, and injury prevention.

Eating Mindfully to Fuel:

For cyclists and runners alike, eating mindfully is crucial to provide their bodies with the best possible nutrition. Understanding food's tastes, textures, and nutritional content helps improve nutrient absorption and digestion, promoting general health and vitality.

Techniques of Visualization:

Training regimens that include visualization are effective mindfulness exercises. Both cyclists and runners may practice their routes or races in their minds, visualizing each pedal stroke and stride. This improves mental clarity and gives students a feeling of security and familiarity with the material.

Paying Attention to the Body:

Being mindful promotes being aware of your body's cues. Exercisers who run or ride may exercise intuitively, modifying their workouts' time or intensity according to how their bodies feel on any given day. As a result, there is less chance of overtraining, burnout is decreased, and a more sustainable training methodology is promoted.

Cognitive Recuperation:

A vital component of every training program is recovery. Techniques like gradual muscular relaxation, yoga, and gentle stretching are examples of mindful rehabilitation. Athletes may speed up their body's healing process and lessen discomfort in their muscles by giving these exercises their whole attention.

Conscientious Stress Reduction:

Cycling and running may be psychologically and physically taxing. Beyond physical activity, mindfulness techniques assist athletes with stress management. Resilience and emotional well-being are enhanced by methods like guided meditation and mindfulness-based stress reduction (MBSR).

Getting in Touch with Nature:

Mindfully immersing oneself in nature may be a life-changing experience for outdoor runners and bikers. Engaging with nature brings a reviving and calming aspect to the activity, whether it is by taking in the ever-changing landscape, feeling the wind, or hearing the noises of the environment.

Inhalation Awareness for Sturdiness:

Maintaining endurance is essential for long-distance running and cycling. Athletes may enhance their endurance performance by controlling their energy consumption, managing tiredness, and keeping a constant pace by paying mindful attention to their breathing.

Physical Systems Benefits:

Practicing mindfulness has a beneficial effect on many bodily systems. By enhancing respiration and the stress response, they support cardiovascular health. Improved self-awareness of the body helps avoid injuries, and stress management strengthens the immune system. Mindfulness cultivates a mind-body connection that enhances cognitive performance and general mental wellness.

In conclusion, runners and cyclists may have a more fulfilling and well-rounded sporting experience by including mindfulness exercises into their daily regimens. Athletes who develop a strong mental and physical bond not only improve their performance but also develop a positive, long-lasting attitude toward their chosen activity.

- **Runners'and Cyclists' Endurance Mental Strategies**

Finding happiness in running, conquering challenges, and reaching objectives are all greatly aided by mental toughness.

For runners, maintaining mental resilience is a complex journey. Using a range of mental strategies may greatly improve one's capacity to deal with the many obstacles that come with running. Here, we'll go into further detail about these tactics to provide runners looking to develop and maintain mental resilience a thorough guide.

Determining Objectives and Visual Aids:

1. Unambiguous Goals: Set SMART (specific, measurable, attainable, relevant, and time-bound) objectives. An organized approach to growth and accomplishment is made possible by breaking down more ambitious objectives into smaller, achievable benchmarks.

2. Visualization: Use visualization exercises to strengthen mental fortitude. Conjure up strong mental pictures of accomplishments, such as finishing a difficult event or breaking a personal best. Visualization helps prepare the mind for achievement as well as boosting confidence.

Positive Self-Talk:

3. Affirmations: To combat self-doubt, build a repertory of uplifting statements. "I am resilient," "I embrace challenges," or "I am capable" are examples of affirmations that support a positive

outlook. Positive self-talk on a regular basis gradually strengthens the foundation of mental toughness.

Presence and Mindfulness:

4. Focused Attention:By focusing on the here and now, runners may incorporate mindfulness into their workouts. Get in touch with your surroundings, your breathing, and the cadence of your steps. Running mindfully improves concentration, lowers anxiety, and raises awareness.

Adaptability and Acceptance:

5. Survival in Adversity: Accept setbacks as a necessary component of the path. Embracing a mindset of flexibility and acceptance allows obstacles to become chances for development. Resilience in the face of difficulty is cultivated by realizing that challenges are a necessary part of every endeavour.

Handling Stress:

6..Relaxation Methods: Include relaxation methods in your exercise and recuperation regimens. Effective techniques for lowering stress levels include gradual muscle relaxation, deep breathing exercises, and meditation. Stress reduction improves mental toughness and keeps one's concentration when running.

The Mind-Body Link:

7. Body Scan Meditation: Practice body scan meditations to develop an awareness of your bodily experiences. By helping runners recognize their points of stress or pain, this exercise cultivates a conscious mind-body connection and enhances general wellbeing.

Building Confidence:

8. Reflection on prior Achievements: Take time each day to consider your prior victories and accomplishments. Remembering successful times

boosts self-esteem and confidence in one's skills, acting as a psychological reserve of power during trying times.

Practice Gratitude:

9. Thankfulness Journaling: Start a thankfulness diary to concentrate on the good things about jogging. During difficult moments, changing perspective may be facilitated by expressing gratitude for the enjoyment of running, accomplishments, or even failures that are reframed as learning opportunities.

Community Aid:

10. Establish Relationships with a Running Community: Foster relationships within the running community. Runners who share their experiences, failures, and triumphs build a supportive network. Strong bonds and a common interest foster emotional fortitude.

Patient and Mindful Pacing:

11. Pacing Techniques: While running, use conscious pacing techniques. Acknowledge the value of patience, especially while participating in lengthy activities. Patience and resilience are fostered by realizing that running is a journey rather than merely a destination.

Restructuring Cognitively:

12. Challenge Negative ideas: During your runs, actively recognize and confront any negative ideas that may come to mind. Through cognitive restructuring, replace self-limiting or illogical ideas with constructive and optimistic viewpoints, which will help you develop mental fortitude.

Difference in Instruction:

13. Incorporate Variety: Mix up your workout regimens to avoid mental exhaustion. Trying out new training plans, surfaces to run on, or jogging routes keeps the mind active, motivates people, and avoids boredom.

Introspective Activities:

14. Journaling: Keep a running notebook for frequent reflection on events, feelings, and

realizations. Writing in a journal helps one become more self-aware, see patterns, and build mental resilience by getting to know oneself better.

Ask for Expert Advice:

15. Mental Coaching: You may want to see a sports psychologist or mental coach for advice. Professional assistance is a vital resource for long-term mental well-being as it provides tailored methods for overcoming particular obstacles and increasing mental resilience.

Athletes may develop and maintain mental resilience by incorporating these all-encompassing mental strategies into their running regimen. Setting goals, talking to yourself positively, practicing mindfulness, and getting encouragement from others all work together to build a strong mental framework that improves performance and makes running a lasting and meaningful experience. The path to mental resilience is a continuous one that calls for dedication, introspection, and a readiness to change and advance.

- **Techniques For Staying Focused On Lengthy Journeys**

For cyclists to not only finish a long ride but also enjoy the experience and ride as well as possible, they must remain resilient and focused. Long journeys may be mentally and physically taxing, from boredom to exhaustion. The use of several methodologies and tactics may make a substantial contribution to maintaining concentration and adaptability throughout prolonged bike pursuits.

1. Establishing Objectives:

Achievable objectives should be set for the lengthy journey. This might include setting objectives for distance travelled, average speed, or certain waypoints. Dividing the journey into more manageable, smaller parts gives you a feeling of achievement and keeps you motivated.

2. Mental Readiness:

It's important to mentally prepare for lengthy rides. Envision the path, foresee any obstacles, and mentally practice conquering them. Having a robust and upbeat outlook before the trip helps you stay mentally strong.

3. Pacing Techniques:

Using sensible pacing techniques helps maintain equilibrium and keeps burnout at bay. Maintain a consistent beat and begin at a comfortable speed. Steer clear of pushing yourself too hard at first, since this might cause early weariness. Maintaining a steady pace helps you save energy for the ride's final sections.

4. Consciously inhaling:

Breathing in a rhythmic and conscious manner promotes relaxation and helps control oxygen intake. To reduce tension and maintain concentration, engage in diaphragmatic breathing exercises. Reducing mental distractions is another benefit of anchoring attention on the breath.

5. Consumption and Hydration:

Maintaining healthy eating and drinking habits are essential for maintaining energy levels. Arrange and bring the right food and water. Maintaining a regular diet of fluids, electrolytes, and carbohydrates promotes both mental and physical stamina.

6. Podcasts and Music:

During lengthy rides, listening to captivating podcasts or music may be an effective distraction. Select uplifting and motivational playlists or material. To be aware of your surroundings, however, particularly while riding in traffic or in uncharted territory, pay attention to the volume.

7. Variability of Terrain:

To avoid boredom, provide variation to the journey. The ride is broken up by hard portions, beautiful scenery, and a variety of terrains that keep the mind active and lower the chance of mental tiredness.

8. Encourage Yourself:

Develop a constructive inner conversation. Motivate yourself, celebrate your successes, and take your mind off of unfavourable ideas. Talking to yourself positively increases mental toughness and makes the journey more effective and pleasurable.

9. Pauses & Downtime:

Plan your breaks wisely so that you may relax and recover. Stretch, hydrate, and refuel throughout your breaks. Short rest intervals help avoid physical fatigue and provide mental refreshment, which makes it simpler to get back on the bike with fresh concentration.

10. Riding in Groups:

Taking a ride with a friend or joining a cycling club may provide beneficial social connection and mutual drive. Long rides might be more fun when there is a feeling of camaraderie among the group members.

11. Methods of Mindfulness:

During the ride, include mindfulness exercises like paying attention to the breath pattern or the feeling of the pedals. By keeping the mind focused on the here and now, mindfulness helps keep it from straying into distracting or unpleasant ideas.

12. Moving Your Body Dynamically:

To lessen physical pain, change postures, stand on the pedals, and use dynamic motions. Periodically shifting positions helps the body stay awake, promotes blood flow, and relieves tense muscles.

13. Establish Milestone Awards:

Set up little incentives for achieving certain benchmarks. This may be a well-planned break, a favorite food, or a beautiful view. By offering material incentives, milestone prizes help the path seem more organized and doable.

14. Plan Flexibility:

Remain flexible in the face of unanticipated events. There might be unforeseen diversions, weather changes, or technological problems. Having an adaptable mentality eases tension and permits changes without degrading the overall enjoyment of the ride.

15. Reflective Activities:

Occasionally consider the trip. Recognize accomplishments, draw lessons from setbacks, and value the experience. Reflective techniques strengthen the cyclist's dedication to the ride by fostering a feeling of fulfilment and purpose.

Combining these methods and approaches results in a more thorough strategy for sustaining resilience and attention on lengthy rides. Cycling may be challenging, but it can also be enjoyable and fulfilling if mental and physical well-being are attended to.

CHAPTER 9

NUTRITION AND HYDRATION

- **SUPPORTING YOUR BODY WITH PROPER NUTRITION**

  - **Nutrition Tips For Runners And Cyclists**

Achieving and sticking to a nutritious diet is crucial for bikers and runners alike. Adequate nourishment not only facilitates peak performance but also enhances general health and recuperation. Let's examine several methods and approaches that might support bikers and runners in creating and adhering to a balanced diet plan.

1. Tailored Dietary Programs:

It's critical to customise dietary regimens based on individual requirements. It is important to take into account variables such age, weight, gender, training volume, and particular objectives. Getting advice from a sports nutritionist may assist develop a customized strategy that fits each athlete's specific needs.

2. Equilibrated macronutrients:

A balanced diet that includes the macronutrients, carbohydrates, proteins, and fats are necessary for both bikers and runners. Proteins are needed for muscle repair, lipids are necessary for general health, and carbohydrates are needed for energy. Maintaining equilibrium between these macronutrients promotes healing and maintains energy levels.

3. Eating Time:

Meal timing is essential for promoting energy during exercise and facilitating recuperation. Sustained energy is obtained by eating a healthy meal two to three hours before exercising. A mix of carbs and protein helps restore glycogen levels and aids in muscle repair after exercise.

4. Strategies for Hydration:

Maintaining enough hydration is essential for bikers and runners. Dehydration may impair performance and raise the chance of being hurt. It's crucial to drink enough water before, during, and after exercise. Beverages high in electrolytes may be helpful for longer exercises, particularly in warm weather.

5. Foods Rich in Nutrients:

Nutrient-dense foods should be prioritized. Vital vitamins and minerals are found in whole grains, lean meats, fruits, vegetables, and healthy fats. These foods boost immunity, promote general health, and facilitate healing.

6. Fueling Up with Carbs for Endurance Events:

Before important competitions, endurance athletes like long-distance bikers and marathon runners might gain from carb loading. This is consuming more carbohydrates in the days before the competition in order to optimize glycogen reserves, which will improve endurance.

7. Snacking Techniques:

Snacking wisely contributes to sustained energy levels throughout the day. Snacks high in nutrients, such as fruit, yogurt, or trail mix, may provide you a rapid energy boost in between meals, particularly if you're exercising hard.

8. Steer Clear of Empty Calories:

It is important to reduce the amount of empty calories that come from sugary foods and drinks. Carbohydrates are necessary, but getting them from whole foods instead of refined sweets promotes long-term health and steady energy levels.

9. Add-ons When Required:

When some nutrients are difficult to get via food alone, supplements may be helpful. Supplements such as vitamin D, iron, and omega-3 fatty acids may be used, particularly if there are particular deficits.

10. Conscientious Consumption:

Observing signs of hunger and fullness is a key component of mindful eating. It promotes a better connection with food and discourages overindulging by encouraging a more mindful approach to meals.

11. Nutritional Periodization:

It's critical to modify diet to fit training cycles. Periodization is varying nutritional intake according to training stages, with more protein during periods of muscle growth and higher carbohydrate intake during intensive exercise.

12. Nutrition for Recuperation:

Nutrition after exercise is essential for healing. Within the first 30 to 60 minutes after physical activity, consuming a combination of carbs and proteins promotes muscle regeneration and helps replace glycogen levels.

13. Testing and Modifying:

As exercise loads or objectives change, so too may the nutritional requirements. It is important for athletes to be flexible with their dietary regimens and adapt as needed to suit their needs in terms of energy, performance, and general health.

14. Learning for Yourself:

Gaining knowledge about dietary fundamentals is powerful. Knowing the dietary requirements unique to their activity may help runners and cyclists make wise decisions and modify their programs as necessary.

15. Regularity and a Long-Term Strategy:

Maintaining a balanced diet plan requires consistency. Taking a long-term approach to nutrition instead of depending on crash diets guarantees long-term results and promotes general well-being.

In conclusion, a mix of individualization, balance, timing, and mindful eating is required to achieve a good nutrition plan for bikers and runners. An effective nutrition plan is one that is developed over time in response to individual reactions and training needs, supporting both short- and long-term objectives.

- **Fueling Your Body For Endurance Activities:**

For endurance athletes like cyclists and runners, properly fueling the body is essential. A healthy diet is essential for maintaining energy levels, improving performance, and promoting recuperation. This in-depth talk will cover pre-, during-, and post-event nutrition as well as a variety of methods and tactics that assist athletes in optimizing their feeding for endurance events.

Fueling for before Endurance Activities:

1. Carbon Filling:

Athletes might stock up on carbohydrates before a lengthy run or cycle. To optimize glycogen storage in the muscles and liver, this entails consuming more carbohydrates in the days before the event. This procedure guarantees that there will be an energy source on hand for the activity.

2. Balanced Pre-Workout Snack:

A balanced lunch two to three hours before the exercise aids in supplying a variety of fats, proteins, and carbs. This may contain healthy fats, lean proteins, and whole grains to provide energy during the endurance competition.

3. Set Up the Hydration System:

Sufficient hydration is essential for peak performance. Pre-hydration is consuming enough liquids in the hours before an activity. Drinks high in electrolytes or water with a dash of salt are good sources of electrolyte balance.

4. Avoiding Foods High in Fiber:

In the short lead-up to an endurance race, athletes should steer clear of high-fiber meals to prevent gastrointestinal upset. These might be more difficult to digest, which could make the run or ride uncomfortable.

5. Bars or Gels of Energy:

Some athletes choose to consume energy bars or gels 15–30 minutes before competition as a rapid and quickly absorbed source of energy. These are handy for fuelling while on the move and provide a concentrated amount of carbs.

Fueling During-Endurance Activity:

1. Intake of Coffee:

Some athletes may see an increase in performance from caffeine. During the endurance exercise, you may strategically eat caffeine-containing gels or chews to increase alertness and decrease perceived effort.

2. Intake of Carbohydrates:

To maintain energy levels throughout the exercise, carbohydrates must be consumed. Sports drinks, energy chews, and gels may help with this. Aim for a steady consumption of 30–60 grams of carbs every hour, modifying according to tolerance and personal requirements.

3. Replacement of Electrolyte:

It is possible for endurance exercises to cause electrolyte loss, especially of sodium and potassium. Sports drinks or electrolyte pills are options for athletes to resupply these vital nutrients and avoid cramping.

4. Actual Dining Selections:

When fuelling up for extended physical exertion, some athletes like genuine food alternatives. This might consist of dried fruits, nut butter sandwiches, bananas, and energy snacks. Trying out several solutions enables one to determine which ones are optimal for personal tastes and digestion.

5. Hydration:

It's important to stay hydrated while going on lengthy rides or runs. Regularly consuming electrolyte-containing sports drinks or water helps restore fluids lost via perspiration and preserve electrolyte balance.

6. Time Management and Regularity:

Consistency is essential for efficient fuelling during endurance sports. Small quantities of fuel should be regularly consumed to avoid energy depletion and to assist keep blood glucose levels stable. During training, experimenting with quantity and timing may help determine the optimal plan for race day.

Fueling after Endurance Activity:

1. Rehydration:

Hydration is still very important after an exercise. It is important for athletes to restore lost fluids with water or rehydration beverages. Including a salt source promotes fluid retention.

2. Consumption of Proteins:

Protein consumption is essential for muscle repair and recovery after exercise. Lean protein sources like chicken or tofu, Greek yogurt, and protein shakes are a few examples of this. Try to consume 15–25 grams of protein in the first hour after physical activity.

3. Refuelling with Carbohydrates:

Restoring glycogen reserves is necessary for healing. Restoring energy reserves is aided by including carbs in the meal or snack after exercise. Choose complex carbs such as whole grains, quinoa, or sweet potatoes.

4. Foods Rich in Nutrients:

A variety of nutrients should be included in the post-activity meal. Including fruits, veggies, and healthy fats meets total nutritional requirements and offers a well-rounded approach to recuperation.

5. Timing Matters:

It's crucial to fuel yourself after an exercise. After exercise, athletes should try to refuel within 30 to 1 hour since this is when the body is most open to absorbing nutrients and replenishing glycogen.

Extra Things to Think About:

1. Customized Method:

People require different kinds of fuel. During training, athletes should try different foods to see what suits them the best in terms of time, quantity, and choice.

2. Pay Attention to the Body:

It is important to be aware of signals related to hunger and fullness. When engaging in endurance sports, athletes should learn to identify when their bodies require nutrition and not ignore their hunger signals.

3. Periodization:

Periodization is the process of adjusting diet to coincide with training cycles. Optimizing performance and recovery may be achieved by modifying carbohydrate intake in accordance with training volume and intensity.

3. Proficient Counselling:

Consulting with a certified nutritionist or dietitian may provide tailored recommendations based on an athlete's unique requirements, guaranteeing they get enough fuel for their competitions and training.

In summary, a comprehensive strategy that takes into account nutrition before, during, and after exercise is necessary for efficient fuelling for bikers and runners. An effective fueling plan for endurance exercises involves experimenting, being consistent, and paying attention to individual requirements. A well-fed body heals more quickly and performs better, both of which are important for long-term sports success.

- **TIPS FOR HYDRATION DURING ENDURANCE EXERCISES**

Drinking enough water is essential for endurance sports since it affects recuperation, performance, and general health. During extended activity, keep in mind the following important factors and advice to stay well hydrated:

1. Prior to Hydration:

Start drinking plenty of water well in advance of the activities. Drink enough water to start the day and keep sipping it during the hours before the endurance exercise.

2. Personalized Fluid Requirements:

Understand that everyone has different demands when it comes to hydration. Individual differences in body weight, perspiration rate, and ambient temperature all affect the amount of fluids needed. Adapt your hydration plan to meet your unique requirements.

3. Balance of Electrolytes:

Sweating during endurance exercises causes electrolyte loss. To assist maintain the body's electrolyte balance, include electrolyte-rich drinks or supplements, particularly for activities lasting longer than an hour.

4. Periodic Hydration Pauses:

Instead of waiting until you are thirsty, include frequent water breaks into your exercise. Preemptive sipping helps prevent dehydration since thirst is not always a reliable indication of one's level of hydration.

5. Timetable for Hydration:

Based on the length and level of intensity of your endurance exercise, create a hydration program. When engaging in lengthier activities, try to stay hydrated by drinking at regular intervals to maintain a steady intake.

6. Water Level Monitoring:

Pay attention to your body's cues. Keep an eye on the colour of your urine: mild yellow indicates proper hydration, whereas dark yellow can indicate dehydration. Moreover, be mindful of any sensations of weariness, thirst, or lightheadedness.

7. Considering Temperature:

Adapt your hydration strategy to the surrounding circumstances. Sweating rises in hot and muggy circumstances and requires consuming more fluids. On the other hand, colder weather could still need drinking water, but perhaps less often.

8. Fuel-Assisted Hydration:

Sync your hydration with fuelling if you plan to use energy gels, bars, or sports drinks throughout your endurance exercise. Drinking liquids in addition to food helps maintain a healthy balance between hydration and energy intake.

9. Hydration After Activity:

After the endurance exercise, drink more water to replace lost fluid. To aid with recuperation, include a mix of electrolyte-containing drinks and water. Estimating fluid loss may be aided by weighing oneself both before and after.

10. Avoid Being Too Hydrated:

Overhydration may be detrimental as much as dehydration. A disease called hyponatremia, which is brought on by consuming too much water, may cause an electrolyte imbalance. Adjust fluid intake based on personal requirements and circumstances.

11. Test and Mistake:

During training sessions, try out various hydration techniques to see which ones are most effective for you. Since each person's body reacts to fluid intake differently, discover a program that works best for you both comfortably and performance-wise.

In summary, proactive preparation, customised tactics, and awareness of the body's cues are all necessary for optimal hydration during endurance sports. During extended activity, maintaining a regular and customised strategy to hydration is critical to maintain energy levels, enhanced performance, and general well-being.

- **Hydration Techniques For Cyclists And Runners:**

For both runners and cyclists, being well hydrated is crucial to performance since optimum physiological function depends on maintaining correct fluid balance. Dehydration may have a detrimental effect on general wellbeing, impair performance, and raise the risk of injury. Let's talk in-depth about hydration tactics for bikers and runners, emphasizing the advantages of each strategy and how to use it.

Runners' Hydration Strategies:

1. Pre- Hydration:

-How to Perform: Make sure you're well-hydrated before the run, preferably in the hours prior. Try to consume 16–20 ounces of water two to three hours before theu run, and an extra 8 ounces 20 to 30 minutes beforehand.

Benefits: By ensuring that runners begin their exercise at the right level of hydration, pre-hydration helps to avoid early dehydration and enhances performance.

2. While Running:

- How to Perform: Depending on variables like temperature and personal sweat rates, drink 7 to 10 ounces of fluid every 10 to 20 minutes while running.

Benefits: Constant hydration helps blood volume, fluid balance, and thermoregulation, all of which are essential for avoiding dehydration and overheating.

3. Replacement of Electrolyte:

- How to Perform: Drinks or supplements high in electrolytes should be taken into consideration, particularly for longer runs. Electrolytes that are lost via perspiration are replaced in part by salt, potassium, and magnesium.

-Benefits: By reducing muscular cramps and hyponatremia (low sodium levels), electrolyte replenishment helps to improve overall performance and recuperation.

4. Hydration After Running:

- How to Perform: Within the first hour after the run, replenish your fluid intake with a mix of electrolyte-rich liquids and water. Make an effort to regain any weight lost throughout the exercise.

Benefits: Drinking enough water after a run aids in recovery by restoring electrolytes and lost fluids, promoting muscular growth, and lowering the chance of post-exercise exhaustion.

Cyclists' Hydration Strategies:

1. Where to Put the Bottle on the Bike:

- How to Do It: Arrange water bottles on the bike so they are easily accessible. Think about using a hydration method that permits you to drink without disturbing your riding rhythm.

Benefits: Easy access promotes frequent drinking, avoiding dehydration and keeping attention on the path or road.

2. Time of Hydration:

- How to Do It: Create a hydration regimen according to the length and level of difficulty of the ride. Drink about every 15 to 20 minutes, taking into account your own sweat rate and the surrounding circumstances.

Benefits: Drinking enough water keeps you energized, keeps your performance from declining, and helps you stay cool on lengthy rides.

3. Gels and Hydration Mixes:

- How to Perform: Especially for longer rides, think about using sports beverages or hydration gels containing electrolytes and carbs. Observe the suggested dilution guidelines.

-Benefits: By combining energy, electrolyte replenishment, and hydration, these products maximize performance and stop the loss of vital nutrients.

4. Rehydrating After a Ride:

- How to Perform: To refill glycogen reserves, eat a well-balanced post-ride meal or snack that contains carbs, electrolytes, and water.

Benefits: Drinking enough water after a ride aids in recuperation, lessens pain in the muscles, and primes the body for further training.

Advantages of Adequate Hydration:

1. Optimization of Performance:

Muscles that are properly hydrated perform better, which improves power production and endurance during cycling and running.

2. Control of Temperature:

- When engaging in vigorous physical activity, being properly hydrated lowers the chance of heat-related disorders by supporting the body's capacity to regulate temperature.

3. Balance of Electrolytes:

Maintaining an appropriate electrolyte balance is essential for nerve transmission, muscular contraction, and cellular functioning in general. Good hydration practices support the maintenance of these equilibriums.

4. Prevention of Injury:

Maintaining enough hydration helps minimize injuries in runners and cyclists by promoting joint lubrication and lowering the chance of cramps and muscular strains.

5. Memory Function:

- Cognitive function is influenced by hydration. Maintaining proper hydration during training or competition enhances concentration, awareness, and decision-making skills.

In conclusion, careful pre-hydration, steady fluid intake during exercise, awareness of electrolyte requirements, and appropriate post-activity rehydration are all important components of efficient hydration methods for cyclists and runners. Athletes may enhance performance, aid in recovery, and preserve general wellbeing by being aware of their unique hydration needs and the surrounding surroundings.

- **The importance of maintaining fluids during lengthy rides:**

It is crucial for both runners and cyclists to stay hydrated throughout extended rides and runs. Maintaining general health, preserving performance, and avoiding the negative consequences of dehydration all depend on proper hydration. Let's explore the significance of maintaining hydration during endurance exercises in more detail:

1. Perfect Physical Condition:

Hydration and physical performance are intimately related. Strength, coordination, and endurance may all suffer from dehydration. Maintaining peak physical performance is critical for long-distance runners and cyclists to meet training objectives and finish events.

2. Control of Temperature:

When engaging in vigorous physical activity, the body produces heat. The main method of cooling down is sweating, and proper hydration is essential for efficient thermoregulation. The body's capacity to sweat is hampered by dehydration, which raises the risk of heat-related ailments including heat exhaustion and heat stroke.

3. Production of Energy:

Maintaining enough hydration is necessary for effective energy generation. A drop in blood volume caused by dehydration might make the heart work harder to pump blood. This in turn impairs energy metabolism and performance by affecting the muscles' ability to receive oxygen and nutrients.

4. Balance of Electrolytes:

Sweat during long runs and rides causes the loss of electrolytes in addition to water. Electrolytes, which include sodium, potassium, and magnesium, are essential for nerve activity, muscular contraction, and fluid equilibrium. It's critical to maintain electrolyte balance to avoid hyponatremia (low sodium levels), exhaustion, and cramping in the muscles.

5. Memory Function:

Dehydration may impact coordination, focus, and decision-making among other cognitive functions. Maintaining mental clarity is essential for safety and peak performance, whether a cyclist is making split-second judgments on the road or a runner negotiating difficult terrain.

6. Decrease in Fatigue:

During lengthy rides and runs, maintaining enough hydration helps to lessen perceived effort and weariness. Athletes who are well hydrated are able to exert themselves for longer lengths of time, postpone the onset of exhaustion, and recover from training sessions more quickly.

7. Cramping Prevention:

Muscle cramps are often linked to electrolyte imbalances and dehydration. Cyclists and runners are prone to cramping, especially during extended activities. Sufficient electrolyte intake and proper hydration can improve overall muscle function and help avoid cramping.

8. System Immune Assistance:

Exercises that take a long time, like long runs or rides, can temporarily suppress the immune system. By guaranteeing that immune cells are adequately circulated throughout the body, maintaining proper hydration promotes immune function. For athletes who often participate in demanding training regimens, this becomes essential.

9. Well-being of the Stomach:

Gastrointestinal problems, such as nausea, vomiting, and stomach cramps, can be exacerbated by dehydration. Staying hydrated may assist avoid pain before and after endurance exercises and is necessary for the digestive system to operate properly.

10. Avoidance of Heat-Related Problems:

Staying hydrated is essential for avoiding heat-related issues including heat exhaustion and heat stroke. It is essential to be well-hydrated during lengthy rides or runs, especially in hot and muggy weather, to prevent the potentially fatal effects of overheating.

11. Recovery After Exercise:

After exercise, maintaining appropriate hydration is still crucial. Rehydrating with electrolytes and water helps the body recover from dehydration, replaces lost fluids, and gets ready for more exercise.

12. Needs for Individual Hydration:

Understanding personal hydration requirements is essential. Athletes differ in terms of body weight, perspiration rate, surroundings, and personal tolerance. Tailoring hydration plans according to these variables guarantees that every runner or cyclist gets what they need.

In summary, the performance, safety, and general well-being of runners and cyclists depend heavily on maintaining proper hydration throughout extended rides and runs. Endurance athletes benefit from consistent and thoughtful hydration habits in terms of both their short- and long-term health and sustainability. Athletes should emphasize drinking fluids and create individualized hydration strategies as a basic part of their training and competition regimens.

CHAPTER 10

RECOVERABLE STRATEGIES

- **The Benefits Of Sleep**

A healthy sleep schedule is essential for runners and cyclists to perform at their best, recover from injuries, and maintain their general wellbeing. Because these endurance sports put a lot of physical strain on the body, getting enough good sleep is crucial to an athlete's training program.

Let's explore the significant role that sleep plays for cyclists and runners.

Body Recovery:

Running and cycling cause tiny strain and injury to muscles. The body starts healing processes during sleep, producing growth hormones and mending broken tissues. Sufficient sleep guarantees effective recuperation, decreasing the likelihood of overuse injuries and enhancing general muscular well-being.

Endocrine System:

Hormones connected to development, stress, and metabolism are among those that are greatly influenced by sleep. Hormone balance is critical for energy metabolism, muscle healing, and stress reduction in runners and bikers. These hormone functions may be adversely affected by sleep patterns that are disturbed.

Improving Performance:

Improved sports performance is closely correlated with getting enough sleep. Cyclists and runners rely on coordination, speed, and endurance—all of which are impacted by getting enough sleep. Research has shown that insufficient sleep may result in suboptimal exercise performance, impaired cognitive function, and heightened sense of exertion during physical activity.

Help for Immune Systems:

Sleep and the immune system are intimately related. A strong immune system is maintained by getting regular, high-quality sleep, which is important for athletes who often strain their bodies to the maximum. A stronger immune system lowers the chance of becoming sick, which guarantees steady training and performance.

Preventing Injuries:

For runners and bikers, fatigue from sleep deprivation raises the risk of injury. Lack of sleep may impair response speed, coordination, and cognitive function, increasing the risk of mishaps or errors made by athletes during practice or competition.

Learning and Memory Consolidation:

Sleep helps with learning and memory consolidation, among other cognitive functions. Training modifications, route memorization, and strategic planning are common activities for runners and cyclists. Restorative sleep improves these cognitive processes, which helps with training and skill development.

Psychological Health and Welfare:

Participating in endurance sports may be psychologically taxing, requiring concentration, fortitude, and stress reduction. Sleep is essential for mental health because it improves emotional resilience, lowers stress levels, and regulates mood. Consistently getting enough sleep helps athletes handle the demands of training and competition.

Perfect Energy Levels:

High energy levels are necessary for prolonged physical exercise. Restoring glycogen storage and making sure the body's energy reserves are sufficiently replenished depend on sleep. Sleep is a must for athletes, and it improves their energy levels both mentally and physically.

Central Nervous System Recovery:

In order to control muscle function and coordinate movement, the central nervous system (CNS) is essential. For runners and cyclists, neuromuscular function, coordination, and agility are critical components that sleep plays in the CNS's healing process.

Control of Body Mass:

For athletes, weight control is a common concern. Hormone balance that governs hunger is impacted by sleep. This equilibrium may be upset by getting too little sleep, which may result in weight gain or make it more difficult to maintain a healthy body composition.

Regularity and Consistency:

Developing a regular sleep schedule improves general well being. Establishing regular sleep schedules enhances the quality of sleep by bringing the body's internal clock into harmony. Maintaining regular sleep schedules enables athletes to optimize the advantages of relaxation and recuperation.

In conclusion, it is impossible to exaggerate how crucial sleep is for bikers and runners. It is an essential element that affects general wellbeing, mental health, physical recuperation, and performance. Athletes are better able to handle the physical and mental demands of their training, which improves performance and increases their chances of long-term athletic success, when they prioritize and regularly get enough restorative sleep.

- **Benefits Of Rest For Recovery In Cyclists And Runners**

Rest is essential for runners' and cyclists' recuperation because it promotes general health, injury avoidance, and performance enhancement. Rest, both in terms of the physical and mental components, is crucial to the healing process. Only then can athletes maintain their training schedules and succeed in their particular fields over the long run. Let's examine the complex function that rest plays in runners' and bikers' recuperation.

Body Restoration:

1. Growth and Repair of Muscles:

Runs and cycles with high intensity cause tiny muscle injury. The body can renew and repair these tissues with enough rest, which encourages the development of muscles and strength. In order to avoid overtraining and lower the chance of chronic injuries, this procedure is crucial.

2. Restoration of Energy:

The body uses its glycogen reserves as an energy source during exercising. Athletes that get enough rest will have enough energy reserves for their next training session. Rest allows these stores to refill.

For long-distance runners and cyclists who exhaust their energy reserves after prolonged exertion, this is especially important.

3. Health of the Joints and Connective Tissue:

Wear and strain may result from repeated impact on joints and connective tissues. Rest facilitates the healing of these structures, lowering inflammation and the possibility of overuse injuries. The body may repair microtrauma and fortify the connective tissues during rest times.

Central Nervous System (CNS) Recovery:

1. Neurological Recovery:

The central nervous system is under stress from intense training. For the central nervous system to heal, avoid burnout, and preserve ideal neuromuscular function, enough sleep is necessary. Enhanced neuromuscular efficiency plays a role in improving running and cycling coordination and gait.

Endocrine System:

1. Control of Cortisol:

Extended and rigorous exercise may raise cortisol levels, which can result in chronic stress. Rest times aid in the regulation of cortisol production, so mitigating the deleterious effects of high stress hormones, including weakened muscles and compromised immune system.

2. Release of Growth Hormones:

Good sleep, which is a necessary component of relaxation, encourages the release of growth hormone. This hormone is essential for muscular development, tissue regeneration, and general recuperation. The best way for runners and cyclists to optimize growth hormone advantages is to prioritise getting enough good sleep.

Preventing Injuries:

1. Preventing Overuse Injury:

Rest is crucial to avoiding overuse injuries, which are brought on by putting certain muscles or joints under constant tension. Insufficient recuperation might make tissues more prone to strain, inflammation, and, eventually, long-term injury.

2. Supercompensation and Adaptation:

It takes time for the body to adjust to the stresses placed on it throughout training. Supercompensation, a period in which the body not only recovers to baseline but also becomes stronger to withstand training loads in the future, is made possible by rest. In order to increase performance over the long run, this adaptation process is essential.

Psychological Health:

1. Avoiding Mental Tiredness:

Constant exercise without sufficient rest may cause mental exhaustion, lower motivation, and raise the possibility of burnout. Athletes may recharge, maintain their passion for their sport, and approach training with fresh concentration when they take a mental vacation during rest.

2. Reduction of Stress:

Stress from training and other stresses in life may compound to have negative impacts on mental health. Rest intervals provide people a chance to unwind mentally, which lowers stress levels overall and encourages optimism.

Coordinated Planning:

1. Periodization :

Periodization is used in training schedules to include rest. In order to allow for recuperation, training cycles usually consist of stages of increasing intensity followed by periods of lowered volume and intensity. In addition to maximizing performance, this strategic planning reduces the possibility of overtraining.

2. Active Recuperation:

Complete inactivity isn't usually the definition of rest. Active rehabilitation, which includes low-intensity workouts like simple cycling or walking, may help to increase blood flow, lessen muscular rigidity, and speed up the healing process without putting the body under undue strain.

In conclusion, rest has a complex function in the recovery of cyclists and runners, including mental health, injury prevention, physical healing, and tactical preparation. Athletes may strike a fine balance between testing their limits and giving their bodies the time and resources they need for the best possible recovery and long-term performance when they understand the value of rest as a crucial component of training.

-Techniques for having a quality sleep for Cyclists and Runners:

Restful sleep is very important for runners and cyclists in order to maximize their training, recuperation, and performance. It is essential for an athlete's general health. Insufficient sleep has been linked to lower energy levels, compromised cognitive abilities, and increased vulnerability to injuries. Fortunately, runners and cyclists may greatly enhance the quality of their sleep by putting into practice efficient procedures and plans.

Creating a Regular Sleep Schedule:

The first step in enhancing the quality of your sleep is to stick to a regular sleep pattern. It is important for bikers and runners to try to go to bed and get up at the same time every day, even on the weekends. Maintaining consistency supports a stronger and more organic sleep-wake cycle by regulating the circadian rhythm, the body's internal clock.

Use Relaxation Techniques to Wind Down:

The body may be told it's time to wind down by including relaxation practices into a pre-sleep regimen. Deep breathing, gradual muscular relaxation, and gentle stretching are a few techniques that may help reduce tension and get the body and mind ready for sound sleep. These exercises may be very helpful for rehabilitation after strenuous training sessions.

Setting Screen Time and Stimulant Limits:

It is important for bikers and runners to watch how much caffeine and nicotine they consume, particularly in the hours before bed. Furthermore, the generation of the hormone melatonin, which promotes sleep, may be disrupted by the blue light that electronic gadgets generate. In order to create a more peaceful sleeping environment, it is recommended that screens be avoided at least one hour before bed.

Establishing a Cozy Sleep Environment:

The setting in which you sleep has a big impact on how well you sleep. Athletes need to spend money on supportive pillows and a comfy mattress. For the best sleeping environment, the bedroom should be kept calm, dark, and cold. White noise machines and blackout curtains may also be used to improve the quality of sleep.

Taking Care of Nutrition at Night:

Nutrition may affect the quality of sleep, therefore athletes should watch what they eat in the evenings. Close to bedtime, heavy or spicy meals may make you uncomfortable, but a light, well-balanced snack might help you go asleep. Although drinking too much water just before bed might cause sleep disturbances, staying hydrated is still important.

Including Calm Sleep Aids in the Mix:

To help you relax at night, use natural sleep aids like herbal teas with chamomile or valerian root in your regimen. To make sure they meet specific medical requirements, it is crucial to speak with a healthcare provider before utilizing any supplements or sleep aids.

Tracking and Controlling the Level of Training:

The timing and volume of training sessions may affect how well a person sleeps. Excessive exercise just before bed may raise cortisol and adrenaline levels, which makes it difficult to relax. It's best to plan your most intense training sessions for early in the day and save your nights for lighter pursuits or relaxation-promoting recovery routines.

Putting Stress-Reduction Strategies into Practice:

For athletes, stress is a prevalent cause that might interfere with their sleep. Using stress-reduction strategies like progressive muscle relaxation, journaling, or mindfulness meditation may help control stress levels. Before going to bed, establish a mental "wind-down" habit that can tell your body it's time to unwind.

Dealing with Sleep Issues:

Cyclists and runners need to be aware of any sleep problems that might interfere with getting a good night's sleep. Sleep apnea, insomnia, and restless legs syndrome are among the conditions that may greatly affect one's ability to fall asleep. In order to treat any underlying sleep issues, it is imperative that you get competent medical guidance and diagnosis.

Timing Exercise and Recuperation:

Periodization is the process of designing training cycles with times of high-intensity exercise and active recuperation in between. Athletes may avoid burnout, lower their risk of overtraining, and improve the quality of their sleep by deliberately including rest and recovery into their training regimens.

Seeking for Expert Advice:

It's critical to seek advice from medical experts, such as sleep specialists or sports medicine specialists, if trouble sleeping continues. These professionals may do evaluations, pinpoint underlying problems, and provide tailored suggestions to enhance the quality of a person's sleep in light of their particular requirements and situation.

In summary, improving sleep quality is a complex process that calls for a thorough strategy from bikers and runners. A good plan must include maintaining regular sleep patterns, learning relaxing methods, setting up a comfortable sleeping environment, and controlling variables like diet and workout volume. Athletes who prioritize good sleep improve their performance and recuperation as well as their long-term health and wellbeing.

• STRETCHING AND SELF-MASSAGE METHODS

Self-care becomes a pillar in the quest of well-being, providing people with an empowering way to revitalize their bodies and minds. Stretching exercises and self-massage are two vital practices that are woven throughout this story. These methods, which go beyond spa treatments and exercise routines, provide people direct control over their own transformational potential and empower them to take charge of their own health.

On the other hand, Self-massage goes beyond simple relaxation; it's a symphony of touch choreographed by one's own hands. It explores the depths of muscle tension, beckoning people to release knots, relax tense muscles, and set off on a comprehensive renewal trip. via the use of focused methods that release particular places of tension or soft strokes that alleviate stress, self-massage becomes a customized ritual that offers the gift of self-compassion via tactile inquiry.

Stretching Methods: Revealing the Flexibility Tapestry

Stretching is a dynamic dance between muscles and tendons, like unfolding a tapestry of flexibility. It's more than just pushing yourself to the limit physically; it's a personal dialogue with your body's potential for movement. By intentionally stretching, people develop a deep knowledge of their own bodies in addition to increasing their flexibility. A closer relationship with one's own anatomy is encouraged by this deliberate investigation of the body's range of motion, which creates a bridge between stillness and dynamism.

Stretching methods and self-massage work well together to invite people to experience a life-changing adventure in the privacy of their own space and time. Through the investigation of touch and movement, a story of self-realization is revealed, enabling each person to take charge of their own well-being. Come along on this journey into the world of self-care, where stretches tell tales of adaptability and perseverance and hands become healers.

Stretching and Self-Massage Methods for Cyclists and Runners for Improving Recuperation and Performance:

It's important to put recovery and injury prevention first since runners and cyclists put their bodies through a lot of repeated and demanding motions. Stretching exercises and self-massage may be a big part of their regimens to help with general wellbeing, muscular imbalance prevention, and flexibility maintenance. Let's take a closer look at these methods, discussing their advantages, particular applications, and easy integration into training plans for cyclists and runners.

Advantages of Self-Massaging:

1. A better flow of blood:

Self-massage improves the supply of nutrients and oxygen to specific muscles by increasing blood flow. By assisting in the elimination of metabolic waste, this improved circulation lessens muscular discomfort and speeds up the healing process.

2. Decreased Knots and Tension in Muscles:

Running and cycling are repeated exercises that may cause knots to grow in the muscles. Self-massage methods that relieve tension, break down adhesions, and ease muscle knots include foam rolling and utilizing massage balls.

3. Enhanced Range of Motion and Flexibility:

Frequent self-massage releases tense muscles and fascia, which improves flexibility. Consequently, this improves range of motion, making it possible for bikers and runners to move more freely and effectively while engaging in their sports.

4. Preventing injuries:

Self-massage helps individuals avoid injuries by correcting tension and imbalances. It protects the general health of muscles and connective tissues, increases the likelihood of strains and sprains, and maintains structural integrity.

- **Ways In Which You Can Do Self-Massage Effectively:**

1. Rolling in foam:

A popular self-massage method that works on a variety of muscle areas is foam rolling. Using the foam roller, runners and cyclists may target particular regions, such as the calves, quadriceps, hamstrings, and IT band, with little pressure. The deliberate, gradual motions increase muscular mobility and relieve stress.

2. Using massaging Balls:

Applying more focused pressure to certain trigger points or muscle knots is made possible by using massage balls. To properly treat tight spots, athletes may lay the massage ball against a wall, along the spine, or under the arch of their foot.

3. Compression Treatment:

Compression sleeves or stockings are used in compression treatment to increase blood flow and lessen discomfort in the muscles. Wearing compression clothing may help with recovery after a run or cycle exercise by reducing swelling and making it easier for metabolic waste products to be expelled.

4. Instrument-Assisted Soft Tissue Mobilization (IASTM):

For more focused self-massage, IASTM equipment like soft tissue scrapers or gua sha may be used. These instruments facilitate tissue mobility by releasing fascial constraints and dissolving scar tissue.

- **Stretching exercises to improve healing and flexibility:**

Stretching is an essential part of every training program for cyclists and runners, and it has several advantages beyond just improving flexibility. In addition to improving flexibility, a well-planned stretching regimen speeds up healing, eases tightness in the muscles, and lowers the chance of injury. We will cover a wide range of stretching methods and regimens designed especially for cyclists and runners in this in-depth conversation.

Dynamic Warm-Up Stretching:

For both runners and cyclists, dynamic stretching is an essential component of the pre-workout regimen.

Dynamic stretching, as contrast to static stretching, includes deliberate motions that allow muscles and joints to reach their maximum range of motion. Stretching like this helps the body warm up, improves blood flow to the muscles, and gets the body ready for the strenuous motions of cycling or running.

Examples of Dynamic Stretching are:

Leg Swings: Take a position next to a wall and slowly swing one leg forth and backward.

Hip Circles: To activate your hip flexors and increase hip joint mobility, rotate your hips in a circular manner.

Arm Circles: To strengthen and increase flexibility in your shoulders, swing your arms in a circular manner.

Static Flexibility Stretching:

Static stretching works well for increasing flexibility and lengthening muscles, while dynamic stretching is best for warming up. When the muscles are heated, runners and cyclists may include static stretches in their post-workout regimen. Muscle fibers may progressively lengthen by holding each stretch for 15 to 30 seconds.

Examples of Static Stretching are:

Stretch your calf by placing one foot behind you, keeping the heel on the floor, and bending forward slightly to feel the stretch.

Stretch your hamstrings by extending one leg while sitting on the floor and reaching toward the toes of the extended leg. This will provide a stretch down the back of your thigh.

Stretch your quadriceps by standing on one leg, grabbing the other leg's ankle behind you, and slowly pulling it toward your buttocks until you feel a stretch in the front of your thigh.

Proprioceptive Neuromuscular Facilitation (PNF):

To improve flexibility, PNF stretching combines static stretching with isometric contractions. This method works especially well for increasing range of motion and encouraging muscular relaxation.

Example of PNF Stretching are:

Stretch your hamstrings with the PNF by lying on your back and lifting one leg. Gently press on the leg for a few seconds with a partner or a band; then, release the pressure and lengthen the stretch.

Using Foam Rolling to Release Myofascial:

Using a foam roller for self-massage is known as foam rolling, or self-myofascial release. It aids in improving mobility and easing stiffness in the muscles by releasing tension in the fascia, the connective tissue that surrounds the muscles.

Examples of Foam Rolling:

Rolling the foam roller gently from the hip to just above the knee will target the IT band. To do the roll, lie on your side with the foam roller under your hip.

Calf Roll: Roll back and forth from the ankle to below the knee while sitting with the foam roller under your calves.

Yoga for Recuperation and Flexibility:

For runners and cyclists, including yoga into the training regimen gives a comprehensive approach to flexibility and recuperation. Asanas improve flexibility, build stabilizing muscles, and provide a calm environment that promotes mental healing.

Yoga Pose for Cyclists and Runners:

Targeting the shoulders, hamstrings, and calves, downward dog increases general body flexibility.

Pigeon Pose: Releases tension from extended sitting or cycling by opening the hips and stretching the hip flexors.

Child's position: This healing position offers a brief moment of relaxation by stretching the shoulders and back.

Stretching the hamstrings and calves while resting on the back provides a mild relaxation in the reclining hand-to-big-toe pose.

The Value of Adaptability in the Healing Process

Since flexibility permits the muscles and joints to move through their whole range of motion, it is essential for the healing process. Muscles might become tired and strained after long runs or bike rides. Frequent stretching helps release metabolic waste products, eases pain in the muscles, and keeps tightness from building up over time and becoming an injury risk.

Adopting Stretching Exercises in the Training Program:

Stretching should be included into a runner's or cyclist's overall training regimen to maximize flexibility and recuperation. The following are important things to remember:

Dynamic stretches are a great way to warm up your muscles and increase joint flexibility before a run or bike workout.

Post-exercise Static Stretching: Set aside time for static stretching after the primary exercise. This keeps the body from becoming rigid and helps cool it down.

Frequent PNF practices: Include weekly PNF stretching practices that target certain muscle areas that might be prone to tightness.

Foam Rolling as Needed: Apply foam rolling often, particularly on days off or when you're feeling tense in your muscles. It could work well as a self-myofascial release tool.

Yoga for Active Recovery: Include yoga classes in your weekly schedule to promote active healing. Yoga not only increases flexibility but also promotes awareness and mental tranquility.

Finally,

A well-rounded training program must include a thorough stretching regimen customized to the unique requirements of cyclists and runners. Athletes can maximize flexibility, reduce the risk of injury, and expedite the healing process by combining dynamic stretches for warm-up, static stretches for flexibility, PNF techniques for increased range of motion, foam rolling for myofascial release, and yoga for overall recovery. Maintaining consistency in these habits improves overall physical and mental well-being in addition to improving performance.

CHAPTER 11

Building a Sustainable Yoga Routine

A comprehensive strategy to improve physical fitness, avoid injuries, and advance general well-being is to create a long-lasting yoga practice that works well with cycling and running training regimens. In-depth instructions on how to design customized yoga routines, the advantages of combining yoga with running and cycle training, and the significance of customizing practices are all covered in this extensive book.

- **Adding Yoga to Exercise Schedules**

1. Incorporating yoga into running training plans

a. Advantages for Runners: Yoga helps runners by treating typical problems including imbalances and tight muscles. Dynamic postures that increase flexibility and joint range of motion, such lunges, leg swings, and warrior sequences, can help to minimize injuries related to running's repetitive nature.

b. Dynamic Warm-up: Including yoga into your warm-up before a run helps your body get ready for the physical challenges that lie ahead. Sun Salutations and leg swings are examples of flowing sequences that improve blood flow, target key muscle groups, and emotionally ease runners into their training.

c. Post-run, restorative postures such as Legs Up the Wall and Child's Pose aid in reducing discomfort in the muscles, releasing tension, and hastening the healing process. This helps keep you jogging on a regular schedule without being distracted by chronic weariness.

2. Including Yoga in Your Cycling Training Routines:

a. Meeting the Needs of Cyclists: Yoga assists cyclists by emphasizing flexibility, core strength, and balance. To address the muscle imbalances caused by extended bike riding, include positions like warrior III, pigeon pose, and cat-cow stretches into your cycling training.

b. Get Ready for the Ride: Including yoga in your warm-up practice before you cycle can improve joint mobility and activate important muscle groups. Bikers may prepare for the demands of the ride by doing poses like Forward Folds and Downward-Facing Dog, which work the quadriceps, hamstrings, and lower back.

c. Pay Attention to Core Stability: Yoga positions that target core stability, such versions of the Boat Pose and Plank, can improve bike posture. This guarantees effective power transmission and reduces lower back strain, improving overall cycling performance.

- **Establishing an Individualised Approach**

- **Customized Yoga Practices for Cyclists and Runners:**

A. For Runner's program:

Dynamic stretches and focused postures are combined to create a yoga program specifically for runners. Stretches for the hip flexors and IT bands, such as Triangle Pose and Crescent Lunge, may help runners who are prone to tightness in certain parts of their bodies.

B. For Cyclists:

To counterbalance the sitting posture on the bike, a cyclist's practice may include hip openers like Pigeon Pose. Including balancing positions like Tree Pose also helps with stability, which is important for bikers negotiating a variety of terrains.

The use of strength-building postures is beneficial for both bikers and runners. Warrior postures help build the quadriceps in runners, while Chair pose strengthens the core and glutes in cyclists, improving their ability to pedal.

- **Advantages of an Eco-Friendly Yoga Practices for Cyclists and Runners:**

1. Injury Prevention:

A consistent yoga practice helps avoid overuse injuries by addressing the muscular imbalances that come with cycling and running. A healthy musculoskeletal system is guaranteed by placing equal emphasis on strength and flexibility.

b. Joint Health: Through the facilitation of a broad range of motion, yoga enhances joint health. Pose variations that include the main joints are beneficial for runners and cyclists as they lower the risk of joint soreness and stiffness.

2. Enhanced Range of Motion and Adaptability:

 a. Targeted stretches: Yoga places a strong focus on stretches that target tight spots in the body. Cyclists get better hip and lower back mobility, while runners have more flexibility in their hamstrings.

b. Effective Movement Patterns: Improved mobility helps athletes move in more effective ways while working out. Running improves stride smoothness, and cycling improves pedal efficiency, so that total performance is maximized.

3. Mental Calmness and Concentration:

a. Mindfulness Techniques: Running and cycling benefit from increased attention during yoga poses that promote mindful awareness. Stress reduction and mental resilience are promoted when mindfulness and meditation practices are incorporated into daily life.

b. Stress Reduction: Yoga's focus on deliberate breathing and meditation help people reduce stress. A more optimistic outlook is facilitated by athletes' ability to control anxiety before competitions and the mental strain of lengthy rides.

4. Enhanced Recuperation:

a. Restorative postures: By encouraging relaxation and lessening muscular pain, restorative postures in yoga improve healing. Athletes may do positions like Savasana after a workout to help them relax more deeply.

b. Circulation and Healing: The blood circulation induced by yoga postures facilitates the transport of nutrients and oxygen to muscles that are exhausted. This speeds up the healing process, enabling bikers and runners to stick to a regular training regimen.

5. Enhanced Stability and Equilibrium:

a. Yoga enhances proprioception, or the body's knowledge of its location in space, by emphasizing balancing postures. For runners to maintain equilibrium on different surfaces and cyclists to navigate uneven terrain, enhanced proprioception is essential.

b. Core Stability: A consistent yoga practice has a strong emphasis on postures that strengthen the core, which improves stability for cyclists and runners alike. For optimal form preservation and effective energy transmission, a robust core is essential.

- Essential Elements of a Long-Term Yoga Practice:

1. Regularity:

a. Consistent Practice: A long-lasting yoga practice is built on consistency. Regular yoga practice has the most positive impact on athletes' training regimens. This guarantees steady gains in mental clarity, strength, and flexibility.

b. Frequency and Length: Individual schedules and fitness levels will determine how often and how long yoga practices last. Shorter sessions integrated more often may have the same positive effects as longer practices conducted less often.

2. The Progressive Method:

a. Gradual Intensity: Using a progressive method, yoga exercises are progressively harder and more intricate. To let the body gradually adapt, athletes should begin with basic postures and work their way up to more advanced versions.

b. Respecting physical boundaries requires paying attention to your body's cues. In particular, while introducing new postures or stepping up their practice, athletes should be mindful of their physical limitations and refrain from exerting too much force. Injury and overexertion risk are decreased with gradual advancement.

3. Mindful Awareness:

a. Body Sensations and Limitations: A key component of mindful awareness is tuning into and acknowledging the body's experiences. Yoga may help athletes become more aware of their bodies, which will encourage them to approach physical exercise with mindfulness and intuition.

b. Breath-Centric Practice: In yoga, mindfulness is centered on the breath. It is recommended that athletes concentrate on breathing in unison with their movements, developing a steady and calming breathing pattern that promotes focus and relaxation.

Printed in Great Britain
by Amazon

829c460c-9906-43da-a86c-8d20ea3479a0R01